Vitamin C Against Cancer

Vitamin C
Against Cancer

H. L. NEWBOLD, M.D.

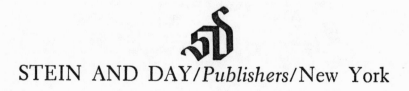

STEIN AND DAY/*Publishers*/New York

This book is dedicated to

My Mother
MARY TEMPERANCE SHERROD NEWBOLD 1898–1974

and

My Father
HERBERT LEON NEWBOLD 1889–1962

Contents

Foreword

The importance of this book by Dr. Newbold cannot be questioned. Vitamin C is one of the earliest specific nutrients to be discovered, and its role in medical history promises to be a far-reaching one. It has long been recognized as an agent which prevents scurvy but in recent years its broader role in promoting life and health has come to the fore.

For all we know at present, vitamin C may be an effective agent in the prevention of hundreds of disease conditions other than overt scurvy. Cancer is, according to evidence presented in this book, such a disease condition.

Dr. Newbold's presentation concerning the advantageous use of vitamin C in the prevention or treatment of cancer and other ailments serves a triple purpose. First, it calls attention to vitamin C itself. Second, by implication, it calls attention to all other nutrients and the whole nutritional team, and, third, it underscores the need for vast research on the part of medical scientists.

If people in general and the medical profession in particular can avoid faddism and quackery and absorb convincing evidence that vitamin C is extremely valuable in the treatment or prevention of disease, this immediately calls attention to the possibility and, indeed, the probability that the same importance resides to a greater or lesser degree in every essential nutrient —every mineral, trace mineral, amino acid, and in each of the other known vitamins. If the nutrients and the nutrient team as a whole work against disease, and if this fact is recognized by the medical profession, it will bring about a profound revolution.

Medicine will become increasingly orthomolecular medicine, in which chemical substances natural to the body are used against disease because of their constructive action, and the use of extraneous, foreign drugs and medicines will be minimized.

One of the fundamental reasons why orthomolecular medicine has such wondrous possibilities is the fact of biochemical individuality. No student of metabolism can, in this day and age, entertain for a moment the concept that all members of the human family are, metabolically, Xerox copies of each other. From a quantitative standpoint there are, among "normal" people, vast ranges of differences in nutritional needs, and the fine tuning of metabolism in any particular individual necessitates meticulous adjustments for the attainment of maximum health. In the field of cancer prevention or treatment, as in every other field of medicine, individuality in metabolism is a vital factor, whether or not we are able to cope with it adequately.

The fact, interestingly presented in this book, that a substantial number of leading medical experts are already thoroughly convinced of the potential benefits of a nutrient, is a momentous one. When all or most medical scientists see that this nutrient (vitamin C) is extremely valuable in maintaining health even under the adverse conditions prescribed by modern life and drug-oriented medicine, it will be commonplace for medical scientists to become seriously interested in other nutrients as well, and a new age in medicine will have arrived.

Roger J. Williams
Professor Emeritus of Biochemistry
University of Texas at Austin
September 15, 1978

Please Read This First

Your friend next door can give you all sorts of advice about health problems without ordering laboratory tests or taking a medical history or doing a physical examination. If his advice works, fine. If not . . . well, it just didn't work out.

However, a physician who is licensed to practice medicine is expected to take the full responsibility for whatever medical advice he gives. For this reason, I cannot directly give any one person medical advice without first ordering laboratory tests, taking a medical history, and doing a physical examination.

Since it is not possible for me to carry out these procedures before allowing you to read this book, I must *insist* that you check with your physician before taking any of the advice I give. Your physician knows you and can judge whether or not the medical advice contained between these covers is appropriate for you.

And he, the man who examines you, must take the responsibility that goes with the medical and diet advice given in this book.

Preface

It isn't often that an entirely new concept of medical treatment is presented to the public within a single book. Yet what you are about to read not only introduces a new concept in medical therapy for cancer, but also establishes a new medical specialty: nutritional oncology.

Onco is the Greek word meaning mass or bulk and has come to mean tumor in our society. More specifically we use it to refer to malignant tumors, to cancers. Oncology simply designates that branch of medicine devoted to the study of cancer. We have oncologists, medical doctors who have as their specialty the diagnosis and treatment of cancer: the surgical oncologist, the radiological oncologist, and, recently, the medical oncologist (who uses chemotherapy to fight cancer).

Now we add a very important fourth member to this team: the nutritional oncologist. This concept is new not only to you, the general public, but also to the medical profession.

I believe all of you, physician and lay person alike, will, after reading this book, be aware of the importance of the new science of nutritional oncology.

Today the general public is flooded with medical information, and people are demanding more and more that they have an active voice in planning their therapy. No longer are they willing to put themselves in the hands of a doctor and blindly follow his advice.

For this reason I have also included chapters in this book on the various forms of non-nutritional treatment available for cancer: hormonal therapy, irradiation therapy, and chemotherapy. More time has been spent discussing the pros and cons of chemotherapy, because the general public is less knowledgeable about this new specialty and because the treatment can make the patient devastatingly ill.

There is no chapter on surgery, since that treatment is rather straightforward and most authorities agree that if cancer can be removed by the scalpel, that is usually the treatment of choice.

It is my feeling that any patient who has been diagnosed as having cancer should have a consultation with all four oncologists: the surgical oncologist, the radiological oncologist, the medical oncologist, and the nutritional oncologist.

Anything less means the patient has a less than ideal chance at getting the therapy best suited to his or her needs.

And the consultation should come before any treatment is undertaken. No matter what the final choice of treatment might be, the nutritional oncologist should continue to see the patient at appropriate intervals.

New York City
August, 1978

Acknowledgments

Marguerite M: Biesele, M.A., William R. Bosien, M.D., Donald R. Davis, Ph.D., Carlton Fredericks, Ph.D., Abram Hoffer, M.D., Ph.D., and Roger J. Williams, Ph.D., were good enough to take time from their busy schedules to read this book in manuscript. I am grateful to them for their helpful suggestions. If the book has any shortcomings, however, I, as the author, must take full responsibility.

In one way or another I have consulted the following and would like to thank them for answering my questions and giving me advice:

Robert C. Atkins, M.D., Private Practice, New York, New York.

Marguerite M. Biesele, M.A., Research Scientist Associate, Clayton Foundation Biochemical Institute, University of Texas at Austin.

George L. Blackburn, M.D., Ph.D., Associate Professor of Surgery, Harvard University School of Medicine, Boston, Massachusetts.

William R. Bosien, M.D., Private Practice, Columbus, North Carolina.

Irwin Bross, Ph.D., Chief Statistician, Roswell Park Memorial Cancer Institute, Buffalo, New York.

Joseph H. Burchenal, M.D., Director of Clinical Investigation, Memorial Hospital for Cancer and Allied Diseases, Professor of Medicine, Cornell University College of Medicine, New York, New York.

Ewan Cameron, M.B., Ch.B., Chief Consultant Surgeon, Dunbartonshire Hospitals, Alexandria, Scotland.

Allan Campbell, M.D., Consultant Physician, Lanarkshire Hospitals, East Kilbride, Scotland.

Glenn Conroy, Ph.D., Assistant Professor of Anthropology, New York University, New York, New York.

Theodore Cooper, M.D., Ph.D., Dean, Medical College, Cornell University, New York, New York.

Donald R. Davis, Ph.D., Research Scientist Associate, Clayton Foundation Biochemical Institute, University of Texas at Austin.

Glen C. Dettman, Ph.D., Director, Oakleigh Pathological Service, Mentone, Australia.

William Etra, M.D., Clinical Instructor in Urology, Mount Sinai School of Medicine of the City University of New York, New York.

Gabriel Fernandes, M.S., Research Associate, Memorial Sloan-Kettering Cancer Institute, New York, New York.

Carlton Fredericks, Ph.D., Professor of Education, Fairleigh Dickinson University, Rutherford, New Jersey.

Robert A. Good, Ph.D., M.D., President and Director, Memorial Sloan-Kettering Cancer Institute Research Professor of Medicine and Pediatrics, Cornell University College of Medicine, New York, New York.

Ezra M. Greenspan, M.D., Clinical Professor of Medicine, Mount Sinai School of Medicine of the City University of New York; President, The Chemotherapy Foundation, New York, New York.

Abram Hoffer, M.D., Ph.D., Physician, Victoria, British Columbia, Canada.

Charles Huggins, M.D., Nobel Laureate, William B. Ogden Distinguished Service Professor (Surgery), University of Chicago, Chicago, Illinois.

Archie Kalokerinos, M.B., B.S., Medical Officer, Aboriginal Medical Services, Sydney, New South Wales, Australia.

Seymour Levitt, M.D., Professor of Therapeutic Radiology, University of Minnesota School of Medicine, Minneapolis, Minnesota.

Jay Patrick, President of Alacer Corporation, Buna Park, California.

Linus Pauling, Ph.D., Nobel Laureate, Linus Pauling Institute of Science and Medicine. (Interview with Jay Patrick.)

William J. Saccoman, M.D., private practice, San Diego, California.

J. V. Schlegel, M.D., Professor of Urology and Chairman of the Department of Tulane University School of Medicine, New Orleans, Louisiana.

Irwin Stone, P.A.-C., San Jose, California.

Albert Szent-Györgi, M.D., Ph.D., Nobel Laureate, National Foundation for Cancer Research, Marine Biological Laboratory, Woods Hole, Massachusetts.

James Watson, Ph.D., Nobel Laureate, Director, Cold Spring Harbor Laboratory, Cold Spring Harbor, New York. (Dr. Watson declined to speak with me. I have learned about his views from secondary sources.)

John H. Weisburger, Ph.D., Vice-President in Charge of Research, American Health Foundation, Valhalla, New York.

Virginia Livingston Wheeler, M.D., private practice, San Diego, California.

Roger J. Williams, Ph.D., Professor of Chemistry Emeritus, Clayton Foundation Biochemical Institute, University of Texas at Austin.

Ernst Wynder, M.D., President, American Health Foundation, New York, New York.

My patient, Rosemary Nay, has taught me a great deal, not only about cancer but also about fortitude and the heights to which the human spirit can soar. Without her this book would probably never have been written. Rosemary, I am grateful to you.

Katheryn Anderson was very helpful during my interviews at Memorial Sloan-Kettering Cancer Institute.

I want to thank Susan Hecht for scouting the libraries for me and for listening to me talk about this book until she must have been bored nearly out of her head.

Introduction

This is the third medical book I have written for the general public. Those of you who have read my previous works might wonder why I have departed from my usual format.

For one thing this is the first book in which I have asked others to contribute. You will find between these covers sections by four Nobel Prize winners, as well as articles by professors from some of the world's best known medical centers. Not even an Arab oil prince could buy time from these men. Yet with this volume you will be privileged to sit across from them and listen to what they have to say about cancer.

You don't want to know only half of what they have to say. You don't want me to decide for you whether the information they give is applicable to you. For this reason I have not tried to edit the information they gave me other than to take out a few surplus "ifs, ands, and buts."

The result may not be literature, but the reader will recognize the ring of truth and reality, which is rare and beautiful in its own way, if not always art.

You will find some material that may seem to be repetitious.

Not so. I have recorded information on the same subject from doctors from different parts of the world so that the reader as well as his physician may discern that the importance of Vitamin C in the prevention and treatment of cancer has become widely recognized.

If you want a perfect piece of art, buy an egg! The intent of this book is to provide information in a way that will enable the layman as well as the physician to determine for himself the validity of the evidence I have attempted to marshal in these pages.

I

Orientation

1

What It's All About

It's amazing how we resist new ideas. Often we must be struck by some strong physical or psychological force before the barriers we build around our minds are penetrated. Once the idea is implanted, however, we wonder why we ever fended off such a simple and obvious truth.

When Newton sat up and rubbed his head after being hit by the apple, he must have asked why he had to wait for a blow to awaken him to the principles of gravity.

It was only a small step from placing a log beneath an object to be moved to making round wheels that would perform like an endless log. And when that first cart rolled by, everyone must have said, "Of course. It's so simple."

For several years I had been aware of Linus Pauling's work using vitamin C to fight cancer. I had even glanced through a paper he had written on the subject. Unfortunately, my head was somewhere else. I didn't really give it much thought.

"Oh, yes," I must have said in my subconscious mind, "another Krebiozen or Laetrile." I had not been an admirer of these treatments for cancer, and doubted that either would ever prove useful.

Then an emotional event happened that changed my whole view on the subject of vitamin C and cancer: The human element entered, in the form of a patient pleading for help. I must admit that when I hear a patient asking for help I must feel the same as a

3

mother who hears a baby cry: I'm uneasy unless I do something to solve the problem. Helping sick people get well was my boyhood dream, and has been my lifetime profession.

"Dr. Newbold," the patient said, "if you don't help me I'm going to kill myself."

Rosemary Nay's First Visit to My Office

The patient, Rosemary Nay (who has given me permission to use her name), was fifty-six years old. She told me that she had been a two-pack-a-day cigarette smoker for twenty-five years and had had a cough for twenty of those years. In May, 1977, she developed a chest pain. When she consulted her family doctor, he took an X ray. As soon as he got a report on the film, he referred her to a cancer specialist, who admitted her to New York's famed Memorial Hospital, the same hospital where Happy Rockefeller was treated for breast cancer and Hubert Humphrey went for surgery after he developed a urinary bladder cancer.

At the hospital they took a biopsy of the cancer by inserting a long needle through the patient's chest wall into the mass they had seen on the X ray. A small section of the tumor was collected in the hollow of the needle. The needle was then pulled out and its contents were removed, fixed, stained, and examined under a microscope.

The doctor gave her the news that every person on earth dreads the most: She had cancer. To be more specific, it was diagnosed as an oat cell cancer of the right lung. Furthermore, the cancer was inoperable, which meant that it was in such a location and so far advanced that there was no hope of eradicating it with surgery.

The death knell had sounded.

They would give her injections of cancer-retarding drugs, referred to more often as chemotherapy, follow this up with cobalt radiation, and hope for 'the best.

4

The whole course would take about two years. Since this was a new approach to cancer treatment (two to five years old), they were unable to talk about long-term results.

The diagnosis of cancer is enough to break the strongest spirit. If we humans are healthy in spirit, however, we have a way of bouncing back no matter how far we're bent. During my nearly thirty-five years as a doctor I have seen parents whose only child died, women whose seemingly healthy husbands suddenly dropped dead, a man whose wife was raped, beaten, and murdered. All of these people worked through their grief. Life wounds all of us, but if we are healthy the wounds close, even though the scars remain. Our spirits are stunned but not broken.

The patient who telephoned me and later visited my office had a spirit that was very nearly destroyed, however. The death sentence had been a great blow, but both she and her husband had been able to withstand that. It was what came next that nearly did her in.

Many people who have been close to a patient undergoing chemotherapy for cancer know how toxic they become, know about the persistent nausea that is often so severe patients are unable to eat. They often lose weight and become so weak that it is an effort for them to move from one room to the the next. A black cloud of hopelessness often descends upon them at this point. They dwell upon the past and mull over in their minds every little negative detail of their lives.

All of us are ashamed about certain things we have said or done, but we who are healthy push these negative memories aside and get on with living today and tomorrow, and tell ourselves we'll try not to make the same mistakes again. Not so with the depressed patient. Those who are depressed grab on to the unhappy events of their past and roll them around and around in their minds. They are too preoccupied with yesterdays to live today and tomorrow.

The drugs used to treat cancer are deadly, and

5

damage all live cells; however, it happens that the fast-growing cancer cells are more sensitive than healthy cells to the onslaught of these drugs. For this reason, the cancer cells are destroyed at a faster rate than the healthy body cells of the patient. The trick is to give as much of the chemotherapy treatment as possible short of killing the patient, with the expectation that many of the cancer cells will be killed outright.

Radiation (such as cobalt) treatment for cancer employs the same principle as chemotherapy. The rays used are toxic for all cells, but more so for the cancer cells. Here again, the hope is to kill as many of the cancer cells as possible without killing the patient.

The patient, Mrs. Nay, was undergoing chemotherapy and had been given cobalt treatments.

When Mrs. Nay first visited me she looked like someone who had escaped from a Nazi concentration camp. The treatment had been so toxic for her that she had lost all the hair on her body, even her pubic hair. Her eyes stared at me from two black holes bored into her skull. Her skin looked as pale and smooth as marble, and was almost as cold. When she walked she looked as if she were moving through water in slow motion.

"I can't take any more," she almost whispered. She was struggling to keep back the tears.

I was certain she was being honest with me when she told me she was ready for suicide. The quality of her life was near zero. Cancer statistics would show she was still living, but they would not mention that her life no longer held any value for her or for anyone else.

"What can you do for me?" she asked. "You're my last hope."

First, I gave her a little speech. I wanted her to know that I was not advising her to abandon conventional radiation and chemotherapy, even though they were making her life miserable. If she was determined

6

to abandon conventional treatment, however, I would be glad to do my best to help her.

Next, I told her about the work done in Scotland by Drs. Linus Pauling and Ewan Cameron. In 1971, these men had begun an experiment with 1,100 terminally ill cancer patients, who were judged to be hopelessly sick and beyond help by any conventional form of cancer therapy. One thousand of these patients were used as controls. One hundred of the patients were selected as the test subjects. The test subjects were matched with the controls so that members of each group had the same type of cancer, suffered from the same stage of cancer, were in the same age group, and so on.

The 100 test patients were given 10 grams (10,000 milligrams) of sodium ascorbate (a form of vitamin C) daily in divided doses. At first the vitamin was administered by vein. As soon as the patients were well enough to take food by mouth, they were switched to oral vitamins.

When Drs. Cameron and Pauling reported the results of this study in 1976 in the *Proceedings of the National Academy of Science,* the 100 patients taking the vitamin C had lived four times as long as the 1,000 control patients who received no added vitamin C.

To be more specific, 90 percent of the vitamin-C-treated patients lived *three* times as long as the untreated patients, and 10 percent of the treated patients lived *twenty* times as long as the untreated patients!

But there was more good news.

While all of the control patients were dead by August, 1976, 18 of the vitamin C patients were still alive!

One interesting patient discontinued the vitamin C treatment after his cancer disappeared. When his growth returned, he started taking vitamin C treatment again. Once more the cancer faded away.

This was probably the best news of all: Not only did the patients live longer, but the quality of their lives was greatly improved.

TREATMENT STARTED

After I finished my little speech Mrs. Nay said she had already made up her mind: She wanted to stop chemotherapy and all conventional forms of cancer treatment and have me treat her with vitamin C.

Before she left the office I gave her the first intravenous injection of vitamin C. I had planned to administer 5 grams (5,000 milligrams), but she developed chills and her nausea became worse, forcing me to stop after only 2.5 grams. I made a note in the chart. Next time I would try her on a brand of sodium ascorbate (vitamin C) that contained no preservative, with the hope that she would have no reaction to it.

I then wrote our directions for her to begin home treatment by taking 1 gram of ascorbic acid (vitamin C) powder in water four times a day, hoping she would be able to keep it down. Also, I placed her on a broad base of vitamins to improve her general nutritional state, instructed her to take dolomite (a source of calcium and magnesium) three times a day, took her off junk foods, and gave her a prescription for thyroid, 30 milligrams daily.

When she returned to see me the next day she was able to tolerate the full 5 grams injection, and reported she had been able to retain the vitamin C and other nutrients.

I might add that for many years I had been giving vitamin C by vein in large amounts for a number of different disorders, but never for cancer.

RESULTS

On the fourth day of her treatments she reported that her nausea had nearly disappeared. She was able to drink large amounts of water and take her supplements without difficulty. For the first time she looked as if she might live. I increased her oral vitamin C to 2 grams four times a day.

8

Because she was making such good progress, I discontinued the intravenous ascorbic acid.

On the sixth day she was greatly improved, much stronger. I added other vitamins and minerals. (In later chapters I will give all the details about supplements and the diet which I recommend.)

At the seventh day she continued much improved, and her vitamin C was upped to 3 grams four times a day.

Thereafter her improvement continued. Gradually her vitamin C was increased until she was taking 36 grams daily in divided doses. Bioflavonoids * were added.

By the time the patient had been on the vitamin C therapy for a month, she looked as if she had been reborn. Her skin glowed pink and healthy. She smiled and laughed while talking to me. She had more energy than she'd ever had, and was working hard and enjoying life.

It's now been four months since I first saw the patient. Her great improvement has continued. The other night she went to Elizabeth Taylor's birthday blast and partied half the night away.

She has had no other form of cancer therapy since seeing me.

Incidentally, when she stopped chemotherapy the doctors at Memorial Hospital told her on the first of December that she would be back begging for more chemotherapy before the end of the month. They were surprised when they checked her over at the end of December and found no evidence of cancer. When they checked her again a few weeks ago the doctors simply shook their heads and said I must know something they didn't know.

I think you would like to hear from Mrs. Nay firsthand about her experiences, so I'm turning the next chapter over to her.

---

* A group of vitaminlike compounds found in nature and associated with vitamin C. They increase the vitamin's effectiveness.

2

Rosemary Nay's Story

The following material is from a taped interview, edited slightly in order to avoid repetition.

ROSEMARY NAY: I was born in a Detroit hospital but spent my childhood in Brazil, Indiana, where I lived some of the time with my grandmother and other times with an aunt. When I was very young my mother died of diabetic complications after having her appendix removed. I attended Catholic schools and then went back to Detroit to attend Wayne University. There I did the usual kinds of things that young girls did at the time. I studied hard, but we had fun at all-night bull sessions and football games and dances. I discovered that American literature was the most beautiful thing in the world. I even tried to write the great American novel.

Eventually I married a young man who was an actor. We struggled along for about fifteen years, and it was just the wrong chemistry for both of us. Then I was a single lady and went to New York in about 1958 and started working for various firms. In 1962 I went to work for a law firm, and I've been there ever since.

I remarried in 1974—a marvelous man, a hippie Jewish businessman who's a Zen Buddhist. He's really a wonderful man, supportive, intelligent, and fun.

H. L. NEWBOLD: What about your work?

My boss, Aaron Frosch, says there is no such thing as a "theatrical attorney." There are only attorneys like him who have clients who work in theater.

Mr. Frosch is a brilliant, magnificent, compassionate man who is volatile and excitable. All the ladies working there are devoted to him and to each other.

One of my first assignments was to open a ledger page called "The Estate of Marilyn Monroe"—in August of 1962. I remember staff tears and pushy newspersons. Everyone loved that little tyke. Mr. Frosch was and is the executor of her estate.

We do many, many personal things. The Frosch office and staff handles all the clients' immigration problems, all of their money, their investment portfolios, their children, the trust fund for each of them and each of their children.

HLN: Did you go to Elizabeth Taylor's birthday party?

RN: Yes. I think of Elizabeth as a "little sister." We understand each other very well. Because of the crowds, I couldn't get near to the little darling at the party. Nobody upstages that lady, and nobody should expect to. Truman Capote danced all evening with Senator Javits's wife. I'll dance with him someday!

HLN: Were you a cigarette smoker?

RN: Yes, I smoked approximately two packs a day for more than twenty-five years, since I was a very young girl. I didn't worry about it, but it did bother me. I coughed a lot.

Last spring I developed an excessive kind of cough. It was a very different kind from the usual phlegmy kind of hack that I ordinarily had. And it was causing chest pains. So a friend recommended that I go see a doctor who was a general practitioner, Dr. Gerson Nonas. The physical examination was within normal limits. But he did the chest X ray and did not like what he saw. So he sent me to Memorial Sloan-Kettering to another doctor, who admitted me to Memorial Hospital on June 3, 1977, and did further diagnostic studies. He is an expert in the field.

There was no question about the mass showing up in the X ray picture. It was about the size of a quarter,

11

and it hadn't been there when I had a chest X ray six months before at the Life Extension Institute.

In spite of the X ray picture they wanted to actually see the cancer cells, so they examined my sputum, which was negative.

Next they put me to sleep and bronchoscoped me—ran a tube down into my windpipe and tried to aspirate tissue growth—but that didn't work either.

Since they were not able to secure material for a microscopic diagnosis, they drilled through my chest with a needle. I was awake for that, because they had to have complete control. It was disturbing, but absolutely painless. They injected Novocain first.

The little needle drill went in to the breastbone. And you could hear it. It crunches. And you didn't dare move or sneeze or blink or breathe, because it was very dangerous.

It took, I would imagine, about an hour, and then later that evening when my doctor was making his rounds, he asked me to have my husband present, which I did, and he explained that it was a malignancy —a solid tumor of the lung.

HLN: What did the doctor tell you?

RN: "Mrs. Nay, I have to tell you that you have a form of carcinoma which we are unable to treat with surgery. If we open up your chest and operate the cancer will spread wider. There are about two hundred kinds of cancer. You are very fortunate in that this is one form of cancer that reacts to chemotherapy. We've had great success with this, about 90 percent * but remember that the program is very young. It is only two to five years old. So we don't guarantee anything. If you wish to take this form of treatment, you'll have to sign a release, the usual sort of thing."

I said I'd like to speak to my husband privately, which I did, and we decided we should try it.

HLN: What did you and your husband discuss?

---

* Dr. Joseph Burchenal, Director of Research at Memorial, says 30 percent to 40 percent, but does not know for how many years the remission lasts.

RN: I asked him how he felt about the chemo-therapy, and he said if you can't have surgery he didn't see much choice.

They told me there would be *some* side effects. Nausea, usually a day or two. Afterwards I realized they talked to me about loss of bone marrow and sus-ceptibility to infection, very high susceptibility, and, of course, loss of body hair and that sort of thing. That kind of cosmetic thing I didn't worry about too much.

HLN: How did you feel when you were told you had inoperable cancer?

RN: I cried a lot. I'm usually a very strong person. I think what is meant to be in life is meant to be, but you also have a responsibility to help yourself. You can't give up. My husband has been very supportive throughout the whole chemotherapy, excepting when he saw what it was doing to me.

I started chemotherapy the next day.

In chemotherapy they administer the drug in your arm, in the vein. I don't know exactly what it is—I think platinum and something else. I don't know very much about drugs, so I didn't try to remember them.

The whole thing took about forty minutes. I felt nothing whatsoever. It was not pleasant or unpleasant. It was just another medication.

But then, oh, wow! The next two hours . . . I was never so nauseated in my whole life, retching from my shoe tops straight up. And that went on for a few days.

They released me a few days after that, and I con-tinued the treatment on an outpatient basis. The protocol was eight days on and three days off, or five days on; I'm not completely sure, I'd have to look in my records. I'm a little fuzzy on that.

I took the chemo with the platinum for about four to six weeks. I was terribly sick for about six weeks. I was working some of the time but not all of the time. But then the nausea got progressively worse. I never really recovered.

On August 3, 1977, I started the cobalt treatment. The protocol is three days on, one day off.

They put you in a room that is lead-lined and you lie on a table and they mark off spaces on your head. By this time you don't have much hair anyway because of the chemotherapy. They paint the area to be cobalted and then bombard it.

HLN: Why did they radiate your head for lung cancer?

RN: They say that nine times out of ten the cancer travels up to the head, from the lung through the lymph system to the head and then down to the lower intestine. They were trying to prevent this from happening, to stop the spread of the disease. They didn't radiate my lungs.

During the treatment you don't really feel anything, but it's frightening to be locked up underneath a big whirring machine that lowers itself down over your body. Then the attendant departs and says, don't be afraid, I'll come back and get you, which they always did, and they tell you not to move, because they only want certain parts . . .

In the beginning I didn't feel any side effects, but soon I became weaker and weaker, especially my knees. I could hardly get up the steps. I'd go to work and it was like being underwater. Every step was difficult. I was depressed, like I was under water too.

I finished the cobalt treatments the end of August or the first of September.

Then they said the next part of the treatment, or protocol, they called it, was more chemicals and drugs. I took three or four injected in the vein, but I was allergic to some of them.

That went on for two or three weeks. Then they want back to the platinum. At that point I told them I needed a rest. I was so weak and nauseated I just couldn't take any more.

November second was my last treatment.

Every now and then I would have another chest X-ray picture taken. They would say to me: "Mrs.

Nay, if that is you, everything is clear. We're really proud of you. Keep up the work."

They couldn't believe that the whole thing cleared up after the first administration of chemotherapy, the platinum. In three weeks it didn't show up any more on the X rays.

HLN: What was the reaction to your request for a rest in December?

RN: They wanted to give me more platinum-14. They said this was a two-year program.

But my husband said I was dying. I was very run-down-looking, skinny and green, and constantly nauseated—constantly. I had circles under my eyes, and I couldn't eat. I was absolutely unable to keep down any food.

Then a friend gave me your book, Dr. Newbold. I had discussed you in my office before with a girl who works with us. I said, I think I have found an alternative answer. And I came to see you. And here I am.

HLN: What was the reaction at Memorial to your coming to see me?

RN: They said they wished me luck but they thought I was committing suicide, and various things like that. They said I would be back begging for more chemotherapy by the end of December; that I was due for a relapse by the end of December. And I said I was seeing Dr. Newbold on December thirteenth.

HLN: What happened when you saw me?

RN: You said that you would listen to my story. You said there were no guarantees, and that your particular system was usually used as a preventive measure, but that you would do your best.

You ordered vitamin-level and mineral tests and blood tests on me. You prescribed a routine of food supplements and megavitamins that was especially high on vitamin C. You also prescribed a "caveman" diet: meat three or four times a day, fresh fruits, fresh vegetables, distilled water, no sugar, no starch.

I got to feeling better and better, and I have had no chemotherapy since then.

15

Now I'm full of energy and ideas, and even my sex life has improved. The nausea disappeared.

I'm taking 36 grams of vitamin C powder a day, divided into four doses. It doesn't bother me at all.

I go back regularly to Memorial Sloan-Kettering for checkups. So far they have not come around to your way of thinking, but they say you must know something they don't know. And I said, I hope so. They can't find any sign of cancer and they are very surprised.

It's now April twelfth and all is well.

At Sloan-Kettering they are just pleased and delighted. They said they don't even recognize me as the same person who came in. They are genuinely surprised and they are all smiles and kisses and hugs.

I feel better than I felt as a young girl. I can run up five flights of subway stairs. I have jolly laughs and great energy, and I work just as many hours as I ever did.

Friends and business clients and acquaintances say, "Oh, Rosemary, you never looked so good in your life, beautiful."

My husband and I are moving to the country, but I want to continue working as long as I can, so long as I feel like it or need to, because I enjoy my job. I enjoy working. I don't think I'd know what to do with myself at home.

HLN: Do you worry about dying?

RN: I never think about it. I just take one day at a time and go along, and I love every single day.

II

Vitamin C Against Cancer

3

Linus Pauling

Fiction has led us to think of scientists as cold, impersonal people whose lives and relationships are ruled solely by their giant intellects. Nothing could be less true about the scientist whose words we are about to hear: Linus Pauling.

Although he is acknowledged to be one of the world's great scientists, having won two Nobel prizes, and although he is seventy-eight years old, there's still something of a pixie about Linus Pauling. His merry cheeks and his twinkling eyes make him look more like a jolly cobbler who sings naughty songs in a light opera than one of the world's great scientists.

I have known Dr. Pauling for almost ten years, and have included him in the dedication of one of my books. My single most lasting memory of him goes back to when I glanced across the room at a scientific meeting and noticed he was holding hands with his wife. When our eyes met he waved to me, gave his wife's hand a squeeze, and turned his attention back to the speaker.

Today Dr. Pauling does much of his work at his home in Big Sur, California, some two hundred miles south of the Linus Pauling Institute of Science and Medicine, in Menlo Park, California. I can think of no pleasanter surroundings. His house sits on the edge of a cliff. The redwood front deck juts out into space. Cool breezes blow from the Pacific Ocean and you can hear the bloom of the waves on the sandy white beach far below.

Jay Patrick is the president of a very successful California corporation marketing nutritional supplements. He was good enough to make the following interview with Dr. Linus Pauling available to me for use in this book.

JAY PATRICK: Dr. Pauling, you've been in Scotland lately, haven't you?

LINUS PAULING: Yes, my wife and I have just come back from our trip to Scotland to visit my associate, Dr. Ewan Cameron. He is the chief surgeon at the Vale of Leven Hospital, Loch Lomondside, Scotland, and for seven years he has been treating cancer patients by giving them large doses of vitamin C. You know that a year and a half ago Dr. Cameron and I published an account of the results obtained with the first 100 terminally ill cancer patients to receive this therapy.

JP: Yes, very encouraging.

LP: Actually, Dr. Cameron first noticed that the patients felt well when they got 10 grams or more, as much as 50 grams a day of vitamin C. They developed good appetites, were full of energy, got up from the hospital and went back to work, and got along much better than with conventional therapy. These were patients who in Scottish medical practice would not have received any treatment except morphine, diamorphine or heroin to control pain.

One of the first things Dr. Cameron noticed was that the patients who were in pain receiving morphine or heroin could be taken off the narcotic drug within five days. He told me about them right here on this deck when he visited our laboratory some years ago, and then he and Dr. Baird published the paper on the effectiveness of vitamin C in controlling pain in cancer patients and also in permitting large amounts of the drug to be taken without having any of the withdrawal symptoms that usually accompany taking a drug addict off a drug.

JP: Yes. Well, they have gone to higher levels in recent months, haven't they, Doctor?

LP: Well, yes. Even at the start Dr. Cameron tried larger amounts than 10 grams a day on some of the patients, and it is clear that the larger amounts are more effective. Twenty or 30 grams a day is more effective than 10 grams a day. But the results are really quite astounding.

JP: Yes. Well, how much do they seem to be extending life?

LP: In the case of the first 100 patients treated with ascorbic acid (sodium ascorbate), these 100 terminal cancer patients were compared with 1,000 matched controls—matched as to type of cancer and the age and sex of the patient. When the paper was published a year and a half ago, it was pointed out that the ascorbate-treated patients had on the average survived more than four times as long after being pronounced terminal than the matched controls. Moreover, a considerable number of them are still alive. I have just gone back to Scotland and have seen some of these patients who, as much as seven years after being pronounced untreatable because of terminal cancer, are still alive and well, with good prospects, I think, of living out their normal life expectancy.

JP: Great. Well, do you now feel that if they were able to get on the higher levels much earlier in life it would make quite a difference?

LP: Oh, yes. I think that the ascorbate would be much more effective if it was taken earlier than when the patient has reached the terminal stage. In fact, we have evidence that the incidence of cancer can be decreased very much by just taking the proper amount of vitamin C, such as 10 grams a day, the amount I take.

JP: That's wonderful. Now of course this is a holistic approach. You and Dr. Cameron are concerned with all the nutrients that they need and the trace elements and so on. Is that correct?

LP: Yes, that's right. I have estimated that on the average people who ingest large amounts of ascorbic acid—say, 10 grams a day, as I do—can expect to live sixteen years longer than those who ingest only the ordinarily recommended RDA amount of 45 milligrams a day. Not only will they live longer, but the length of the period of really good life, real well-being, can be extended by sixteen years.

In addition, there will be benefits from taking some other dietary supplements, other vitamins, cutting down on the intake of sugar, exercising, and not smoking. These methods of improving one's health offer great possibilities.

JP: Doctor, could we talk about your work with cholesterol? Isn't it a great myth that is being propounded lately?

LP: I think it is a myth that one should decrease the amount of cholesterol that is eaten. Eggs, for example, are a very good food, and I don't think we should be restricted in eating them. You know every human being manufactures cholesterol in the cells of his own body, 2 or 3 grams a day, and then on top of that he gets some dietary cholesterol, 250 milligrams, a quarter of a gram, in an egg.

I think there is a feedback mechanism such that if you increase the amount that you ingest then you don't synthesize so much. And there are observations showing that people that have a high dietary intake of cholesterol have only the same level of cholesterol in their body as those on a low dietary intake.

Dr. Spittle [of Great Britain] pointed out that a person without athrosclerosis, an ordinary person, who ingests a gram or more of vitamin C per day has a decreased level of cholesterol in the blood, and Dr. Ginter [of Czechoslovakia] found the mechanism for this effect, which is that the vitamin C increases the rate at which the cholesterol is broken down and eliminated as bile acids. So vitamin C is beneficial to heart patients, too, and it helps to clear the cholesterol-calcium plaques that form in blood vessels.

I don't believe that vitamin C is a special anticancer wonder drug. I think that vitamin C works against cancer by bolstering the body's natural protective mechanisms in a number of different ways. The various immune mechanisms, for example. This means that it can be effective also against heart disease and against

22

the various infectious diseases, and not only infectious diseases but degenerative diseases. It improves the health generally when it is taken in the proper amounts.

JP: Would you say then that vitamin C is about the only true panacea? That that's where we can use that word?

LP: I believe that vitamin C is a panacea substance that will benefit you no matter what is wrong with you. It is a special sort of substance. It is a prototype of the agents of orthomolecular medicine, the substances that are normally present in your body, whose concentrations can be varied in order to improve health and give greater resistance to disease.

JP: Well, that's wonderful. That certainly helps bring us up-to-date, Dr. Pauling. I want to thank you very much for spending the time to talk this over with me.

4

Ewan Cameron

On a shirtsleeve-warm, bright April day I drove the eighteen miles east from Glasgow to Loch Lomondside, a village bordering Loch Lomond—the lake made famous by the Scottish poet Robert Burns—where the Vale of Leven District General Hospital sits perched on the top of a hill.

On the way I passed fascinating shops with signs advertising such things as grass machines (lawn mowers) and sign writers (sign painters). When I stopped once or twice to ask directions I had to strain to understand the heavy Scottish brogue. I found the apple-cheeked people friendly and eager to help a stranger.

After climbing the winding road to the top of a hill, I found what looked to be at first sight a new, modern small hospital. I say at first sight because I had come upon the maternity section at the top of the hill. This building was well kept and was by far the largest in the group making up the hospital.

To the right of the maternity building sat the much smaller medical-surgical part of the hospital. Apparently this had been built earlier than the maternity wing, for it showed signs of wear. The vinyl-tile floor covering the entryway had been worn through. The waiting room was quite small. Since there was no information desk, I had to wander around to the emergency room to get directions. A nurse's assistant

was good enough to take me up to Mr. Cameron's
office.*

My Talk with Mr. Cameron, Chief of Surgery

Mr. Cameron, apparently in his sixties, was a tall,
quiet-mannered man with large features and a solid
chin. His shaggy dark eyebrows were in dramatic contrast to his full head of gray hair. He looked like a
kind, successful grandfather who had kept his figure,
his wit, and his wits.

I found he shared a small, rather bare office with his
secretary. During the whole interview we were sere-
naded from below by the sound of a jackhammer
blasting concrete away to make room for a new operating theater (operating room to Americans).

When I pulled out my tape recorder and indicated
that I would like him to hold the mike, Mr. Cameron
recoiled and explained he didn't like "those kind of
things."

I had traveled four thousand miles to spend an hour
with him. I certainly didn't want to turn him off at
this point, but I was also determined to get the best
possible interview. As a compromise, I simply turned
on the mike and held it in his direction while he
talked; I couldn't help thinking of the blanks my
secretary would have in her notes when she typed
them up.

Although Mr. Cameron is a Scotsman bred (Isle of
Lismore, off the West Coast of Scotland, population
110), he has an upper-class English accent and thus,
typically, speaks without doing anything so vulgar as

---

* In the British Isles physicians ordinarily earn a Bachelor
of Medicine and a Bachelor of Surgery degree upon gradua-
tion from medical school, and are called "Doctor" only as a
courtesy. Once a "doctor" has taken his postgraduate training
and is a qualified surgeon he is addressed as "Mister" rather
than as "Doctor," which I suppose is a sort of reverse snob-
bery.

25

opening his mouth. The effect has been described as sounding as though they are talking while holding a mouthful of mush.

As if to prove that the gods were all against me on this day, the jackhammer down below increased in fury and was soon joined by a loud popping, gurgling sound from the hospitable coffeepot on a nearby table.

Mr. Cameron told me that his interest in vitamin C therapy for cancer went back to 1966, when his book putting forth some of his views about cancer was published. One of the things that people seemed to forget about cancer is that in treating it, doctors are not treating something that happened to the patient from outside. An influenza virus, for example, invades the body from outside, and we treat the body in an attempt to do away with the virus. But in the case of cancer cells we are treating something that has gone wrong in the body itself, and in this sense what is happening is not foreign to the body. Certain body cells start reproducing in an uncontrolled manner and invade the other tissues; eventually the patient dies.

Mr. Cameron feels that we pay far too little attention to the individual patient's resistance to cancer and do too little to help improve that resistance. Many people, for example, are exposed to herpes simplex Type 2 viruses, which are known to produce cancer, and yet a relatively small percentage of people develop cancer. The question is, why do some people resist cancer and others succumb to it? Doctors should spend more time improving the resistance of patients to cancer and should approach the whole problem from that standpoint.

For example, it is all well and good to treat a patient with pneumonia by using penicillin and other antibiotics; however, if the patient had had proper nutrition, he might not have developed the pneumonia in the first place, and certainly it is more important in medicine to prevent disease than it is to treat it after it has already developed.

ON DRUGS FOR CANCER

Mr. Cameron feels that cytotoxic drugs (chemotherapy) pose a great stress on cancer patients and may in fact lower their natural resistance to fight the disease. He points out that the results of chemotherapy in treating cancer patients are really unknown at this time. He feels it is certainly a mistake to push chemotherapy in the treatment of cancer to the bitter end. For example, some physicians administer chemotherapy to a patient up until the day he dies, presumably because the patient's feeling that something is being done for him helps his morale. In fact, chemotherapy is a devastating therapy, and not only may not prolong patients' lives but also may make the cancer patients feel miserable during the last months of their lives, when these months might otherwise possibly have been productive months during which the cancer patient could have felt relatively well.

THE BODY CEMENT

Mr. Cameron points out that there is a natural propensity for body cells to reproduce. For instance if you remove cells from a person and place them in a nutrient broth in a temperature-controlled laboratory situation, they reproduce quite readily. Once outside the human body, there is nothing to hold them in check. Cells in the human body reproduce readily also —when one has an injury, such as a cut, the surrounding body cells quickly begin reproducing and heal the injury—but only, in the normal course of events, while there is a specific need for them to do so. When the cut has healed the cells stop reproducing. The point Mr. Cameron makes is that the collagen (the cement) in the human body holds cells in check and keeps them from reproducing in an uncontrolled manner.

He notes that in scurvy the body cells tend to lose their ability to hang together because of a loss of collagen. He feels it is this same cement which holds cells in check and keeps them from reproducing in a haphazard manner.

More technically, Mr. Cameron views malignant disease as a disorder of the hyaluronidase complex. The body cells are enmeshed in collagen, made up of glycosaminoglycans. If anything interferes with these glycosaminoglycans, the cells lose their cohesion and are free to invade other tissue.

Collagen (or glycosaminoglycans) can undergo depolymerization by a body enzyme known as hyaluronidase. This enzyme is held in check by a substance called PHI (physiological hyaluronidase-inhibitor). This PHI needs vitamin C for its manufacture. If the body's vitamin C levels are too low, the PHI may not be present in adequate amounts to inhibit the destruction of the collagen by the enzyme, and the cells thus would be free to reproduce in a haphazard way, as in cancer.

Mr. Cameron has measured the vitamin C body levels both in the serum and in the white blood corpuscles of many hundreds of cancer patients and found that they are low in vitamin C. Parenthetically, it is interesting that surgery, X ray and cobalt treatment, as well as cancer chemotherapy, all lower the patient's vitamin C levels.

Mr. Cameron points out that since malignant cells have the ability to destroy the collagen that surrounds them, they get into the lymphatic system and the bloodstream and spread through the body.

Rapidly growing cancer cells require a great deal of nutrient substances such as vitamins and minerals in order to keep reproducing. They tend to rob the body of these substances and thus to lower the body's resistance even further.

He points out that the only difference between cancer cells' proliferation and the proliferation of cells in wound healing is that the wound-healing cells are contained and stopped from reproducing after they have served their purpose—stopped by the collagen in which they are embedded. With cancer cells, on the other hand, the collagen is not of sufficient quality to hold them in check. The quality of the collagen can be improved by administering large amounts of vitamin C.

DID VITAMIN C HELP PATIENTS WITH CANCER?

Mr. Cameron spoke briefly about the research project carried out by him and Linus Pauling from 1971 to 1976. (See Appendix A.)

Eleven hundred patients suffering from terminal cancer were used in the project. One thousand cancer patients served as controls. These were matched as to type of cancer, stage of cancer, age of patients, etc., with the 100 patients who were in the treatment group.

Please remember that all 1,100 patients were terminally ill and had been judged by several doctors to be untreatable by standard methods, such as chemotherapy, radiation, or surgery.

Each patient had cancer proven by biopsy.

The 100 treated patients were given 10 grams of vitamin C daily in divided doses. The 1,000 control patients were not given any vitamin C beyond what they got in their normal diet.

The results were as follows:

1. Ninety percent of the 100 patients treated with vitamin C lived three times as long as the 1,000 untreated patients.

2. Ten percent of the 100 treated patients lived twenty times as long as the untreated patients.

3. The treated patients had far less pain, were happier, and led more productive lives than the untreated patients.

4. At the end of the research project all of the 1,000 untreated patients were dead. Eighteen of the treated patients were still alive.

Who can argue with the results from such a well-controlled study?

Mr. Cameron pointed out that of the original 100 patients treated, six patients were still living (as of

1978). The one who has been alive longest is a woman with breast cancer who was told seven years ago that she was judged terminally ill and there was no treatment likely to be of any benefit to her. She has been on vitamin C constantly at 10 gram level and remains in good health. He pointed out that the patients tended to be in the older age group and that some of the vitamin-C-treated patients died from causes other than cancer.

OTHER VITAMINS FOR CANCER PATIENTS

When asked if he was still treating cancer patients with 10 grams of sodium ascorbate, Mr. Cameron said he was. He has difficulty getting patients to tolerate more than 10 grams daily, and that lack of toleration has been one of the limiting factors and keep him from pushing vitamin C to higher levels. He feels that some patients who do not benefit from 10 grams daily of vitamin C might well benefit from much higher levels of the vitamin.

Mr. Cameron uses either the fine-powder form—rather than the coarse-granulated, which looks like sugar—of ascorbic acid, sodium ascorbate, or calcium ascorbate, depending on which of the three his patients can best tolerate. The sodium ion is contraindicated in people with high blood pressure or some heart trouble, kidney disorders, and so forth.

Mr. Cameron stated that his patients usually take the vitamin C after eating.

Mr. Cameron does not use bioflavonoids along with vitamin C, though he thinks it might be a good idea.

I suggested that since he was talking about resistance to cancer, it would seem appropriate to give other vitamins and a well-balanced diet to his patients in order to increase their resistance. He agreed, but he had not pursued the idea because he was particularly interested in vitamin C and felt that to mix in other vitamins would alter his research program, which is aimed at discovering whether vitamin C has any effect on prolonging the life of patients with cancer. He stated that his patients were on a good diet, but I found it to be only the ordinary hospital diet, which I myself consider extraordinarily inadequate, mainly because of the processed foods which it contains and the high carbohydrate level.

Mr. Cameron admitted that maybe the most basic reason he has not used other vitamins and minerals nor stressed diet more is simply because he is not sophisticated in the field of human nutrition.

CHEMOTHERAPY FOR CANCER

The question arose as to whether chemotherapy could be used with vitamin C therapy. Mr. Cameron reminded me that chemotherapy was generally not as popular in the British Isles as in the United States. It was his feeling that some cancer patients would be better off not treated with chemotherapy, because it was problematical whether or not it would prolong their lives; more important, chemotherapy made patients much more miserable while they did live because of the weakness, depression, nausea, headaches, and other symptoms that accompany the treatment. He said he believed it was a mistake in the United States to have a policy of treating cancer patients with chemotherapy up until the day they died.

Mr. Cameron pointed out that patients who are receiving vitamin C in large doses tolerate chemotherapy with much less discomfort. Two visiting Japanese physicians had told him that they gave the patients intravenous chemotherapy and followed it later with intravenous vitamin C, and were pleased with the results on this regime.

I brought up the fact that vitamin C is a strong detoxifier. For example, Antabuse is used to keep alcoholics from drinking alcohol. When patients taking Antabuse drink alcohol, they become very nauseated, have a fast-beating heart, get a headache, and become quite ill. It is well known, however, that large amounts of vitamin C will protect the patients from this effect of Antabuse and thus effectively cancel out its use.

I asked if a patient receiving chemotherapy would feel much better if the chemotherapeutic agent was detoxified by vitamin C—and would vitamin C protect not only the patient's healthy cells but also the cancer cells from chemotherapy?

Mr. Cameron said that this was a very real possibility but that no one knew the answer at present. From a clinical standpoint, he had not observed that the patients who took chemotherapy and ascorbic acid responded less well to the chemotherapy. He did not think that ascorbic acid was blocking the chemotherapy. If it did block it, then the ascorbic acid was more than making up for any loss of chemotherapeutic effectiveness.

He concluded that chemotherapy plus ascorbic acid was not contraindicated.

Did he feel that ascorbic acid was effective in preventing cancer? Mr. Cameron said that since the vitamin helped contain and cure cancer, then quite obviously its use in preventing cancer was clearly indicated. He pointed out that everyone is exposed to viruses, X ray and ultraviolet radiation, and carcinogenic chemicals—all of which produce cancer in some people—but not everyone develops cancer, so there must be a difference in resistance to it from one person to the next. Vitamin C and other vitamins plus proper nutrition almost surely play a part in this resistance.

An Extra Benefit from Vitamin C

He commented on the fact that in his experience HDL (high-density lipoprotein) were elevated by taking large amounts of vitamin C. High-density lipoproteins have been found to be more highly correlated than cholesterol levels with cardiovascular diseases such as coronary artery disease and strokes. Unlike cholesterol, however, the *higher* the HDL level, the less likelihood of cardiovascular disease. Mr. Cameron felt that, if for no other reason than to elevate the HDLs, people should take ascorbic acid in generous amounts. (Incidentally, my patients also have an elevated HDL with administration of megadoses of ascorbic acid.)

Mr. Cameron himself takes only 1 gram a day of vitamin C.

I might point out that the second and third fingers of Mr. Cameron's right hand are stained quite brown from smoking cigarettes. He seemed embarrassed when he admitted to being a cigarette smoker. His smoking seemed extraordinary to me in view of his great in-interest in cancer.

When Mr. Cameron was asked if his colleagues in the medical profession gave him any difficulty over his use of vitamin C, he stated that most of them had at first looked on it as a harmless escapade on his part. They had no idea that such a common substance as vitamin C could possibly be of any assistance in cancer. However, they gradually changed their attitude about it, and a number of physicians in Scotland are now using it for their cancer patients.

I remarked on how difficult it was to get a new idea implanted in society's collective thinking and that I thought the general public would develop a greater interest in the use of vitamin C for cancer if I could interview and write about some of his patients who had taken his new treatment. Mr. Cameron agreed that the personal element was important but that he would be very much against patients being interviewed, because in Britain it was common practice not to tell patients that they had cancer.

Mr. Cameron then began to tell me about several of his patients.

The first was a truck driver in his forties who was admitted to the hospital complaining of fever, weakness, and nausea. A chest X ray showed the invasion of cancer in the lung. He also had large lymph nodes in his neck which were cancerous. A biopsy proved the diagnosis: reticulum cell sarcoma.

This patient was scheduled to be transferred to a cancer treatment center specializing in chemotherapy.

However, they were short of beds at that hospital and decided to give preference to a younger patient, a man in his thirties with three children.* They anticipated having room for Mr. Cameron's patient several weeks later.

In the meantime, since the patient was inoperable, Mr. Cameron decided to start him on vitamin C. Accordingly, he was given 10 grams a day of sodium ascorbate in divided doses. Mr. Cameron reported that the response was remarkable. In four or five days the glands in the patient's neck disappeared, the chest X ray cleared up, the patient lost his fever, his strength returned, he was eating well, and by the end of the week there was no evidence of cancer. Because of the excellent response, it was decided not to start the patient on chemotherapy after all.

The patient returned to work and continued to take his vitamin C for a number of months. However, human nature being what it is, the patient decided he was doing so well that he could stop taking his vitamin C. Soon after he discontinued the vitamin, his symptoms began returning. He got weak again, his nausea returned, he started losing weight, and the glands in his neck swelled once more. On his readmission to the hospital, a chest X ray showed cancer invasion. Another biopsy was taken from one of the lymph nodes of his neck. Once more the diagnosis of cancer was confirmed.

Accordingly, this patient was again started on vitamin C, 10 grams daily. Again all the patient's symptoms disappeared, though somewhat more slowly than before. The lymph nodes in his neck gradually subsided, and another chest X ray revealed that the cancer had disappeared from his lungs.

This was several years ago. The patient remains in good health and continues to take his vitamin C. He returned to work and still drives a truck from Glasgow to London, delivering Rolls-Royce engines.

---

* Does this tell us something about their system of socialized medicine?

Mr. Cameron then told me about another patient, sixty-one years old and terminally ill from cancer when his vitamin C therapy was begun. This patient had a very good remission from his symptoms. He not only got out of his hospital bed but returned home and lived a very active life for two years. During this time he was active as a yachtsman, sailing in races all over European waters. He even reduced his golf score by three points, a very important victory for a Scotsman. (Golf was invented in Scotland.) Because of the nature of his business, he traveled extensively around the world in the following two years. He felt very good. At the end of the two-year period his cancer suddenly returned. An increase in his vitamin C dosage did not help. He had a very rapid downhill course, and died in about two weeks.

Mr. Cameron said that this patient illustrated a point which he had repeatedly observed in terminally ill cancer patients treated with vitamin C: Not only were their lives prolonged, but the *quality* of their lives was greatly improved during the time that they did live. They felt much better and were much more active. Their spirits were better. When these patients came to the end of the road they went downhill very rapidly, and died quickly without the usual suffering.

Mr. Cameron stated that patients who were terminally ill with cancer and taking large amounts of heroin, morphine, or other painkillers most commonly were able to get off these drugs. With vitamin C treatment the cancer stopped invading the bone, and thus the pain ceased.

Even though some of these patients may not have lived any longer than patients without vitamin C, they had a much more comfortable life during their terminal illness. Mr. Cameron stated that this freedom from pain was a most important point which should be borne in mind by all physicians treating terminally ill cancer patients.

Mr. Cameron pointed out that under stress animals manufacture vitamin C. For example, if a goat is subjected to stressful conditions its body will make enormous amounts of vitamin C. There is hardly any question that cancer is a stressful condition. If human beings could manufacture their own vitamin C, they would do so in large amounts at the onset of cancer. Since we are one of the few animals whose bodies cannot make their own vitamin C, it behooves us to take it in large amounts when we are in stressful conditions, such as suffering from cancer.

We discussed the possible difficulties with sodium in the sodium ascorbate. Mr. Cameron said that some people do have trouble with the sodium ion, particularly older people who may be in cardiac failure, in kidney failure, or have high blood pressure, and that some of them are given the straight ascorbic acid powder and others the calcium ascorbate powder.

Mr. Cameron was not aware of physicians in the United States who might be using vitamin C for terminal cancer patients, although he has received numerous letters from patients in the States asking about the treatment.

I asked Mr. Cameron what he would do if he had cancer.

He said he would have it cut out if possible. Otherwise, he did not think he would take chemotherapy, because it made people so ill and seemed to rob them of the quality of the last months of their life; rather, he would go on massive amounts of vitamin C, in the same way he treated his patients. He pointed out that he feels too much chemotherapy is used, and used too late, in the treatment of cancer. It's a matter of doctors having to doctor, just as government leaders have to govern. There is a tendency for all people to run their profession into the ground, to the exclusion of the over-all benefit to mankind.

I told Mr. Cameron about a prominent personality in New York who took several years to die of cancer, and had received chemotherapy all the way to his deathbed. He had smoked four packs of cigarettes a day. Since each cigarette destroys up to about 25 milligrams of vitamin C, and since this patient did not take any supplements of vitamin C whatsoever, one can imagine what his vitamin C level must have been. He was on a large quantity of opiates for pain. In my view, this was an unthinkable way to manage cancer. The patient lived out his last years in utter misery.

After our conversation, Mr. Cameron and I went outside for a picture-taking session.

He said I looked as if I had some Scotch blood in me, and I told him my maternal grandfather's ancestors were Scotch.

"Sherrod. Is that a Scotch name?" I asked.

"Oh, yes," he replied. "Sherrod would be from the eastern part of Scotland."

We shook hands and I drove back to my hotel in Glasgow, carefully reminding myself to stay on the left side of the road and feeling as if my anxiety called for an extra amount of vitamin C every time I rounded a curve, half expecting to meet another car head-on.

I couldn't help thinking about the important work Mr. Cameron was doing. Here, in a very modest hospital, using only a few hundred dollars for the entire research program, and largely unknown to the world at large, he had made a very important step forward in the battle against cancer.

I felt that his research was far and away more important than much that was done in the great skyscraper, gleaming glass-and-concrete medical centers in America with all their millions of dollars of government subsidy.

BIBLIOGRAPHY

Cameron, Ewan. "Biological Function of Ascorbic Acid and the Patho-genesis of Scurvy," *Medical Hypotheses*, vol. 2, pp. 154–163, 1976.
—— *Hyaluronidase and Cancer*. Oxford and New York: Pergamon Press, Inc., 1966.
—— "Vitamin C," *British Journal of Hospital Medicine*, vol. 13, p. 511, 1975.

―― and Gillian Baird. "Ascorbic Acid and Dependence on Opiates in Patients with Advanced Disseminated Cancer," *International Research Communications Systems,* August, 1973.

Cameron, Ewan, and Allan Campbell, "The Orthomolecular Treatment of Cancer II. Clinical Trial of High-Dose Ascorbic Acid Supplements in Advanced Human Cancer," *Chemico-Biological Interactions,* vol. 9, pp. 285–315, 1974.

―― and Thomas Jack. "The Orthomolecular Treatment of Cancer III. Reticulum Cell Sarcoma: Double Complete Regression Induced by High-Dose Ascorbic Acid Therapy," *Chemico-Biological Interactions,* vol. 11, pp. 387–93, 1975.

Cameron, Ewan, and Linus Pauling, "Ascorbic Acid and the Glycosamino-glycans: An Orthomolecular Approach to Cancer and Other Diseases," *Oncology,* vol. 27, pp. 181–92, 1973.

―― "The Orthomolecular Treatment of Cancer I. The Role of Ascorbic Acid in Host Resistance," *Chemico-Biological Interactions,* vol. 9, pp. 273-83, 1974.

―― "Supplemental Ascorbate in the Supportive Treatment of Cancer I. Prolongation of Survival Times in Terminal Human Cancer," *Proceedings of the National Academy of Sciences U.S.A.,* vol. 73, pp. 3685–89, 1976.

Cameron, Ewan, and Douglas Rotman, "Ascorbic Acid, Cell Proliferation and Cancer," *Lancet,* vol. 1, p. 542, 1972.

Allan Campbell

One of the physicians in Scotland who has worked with and collaborated with Mr. Cameron is Allan Campbell, M.D., F.R.C.P. Dr. Campbell is a physician; unlike most physicians in the British Isles, he holds an M.D. degree rather than a Bachelor's degree. This means he wrote an M.D. thesis.

I telephoned Dr. Campbell on late notice. He was gracious enough to cancel two meetings and travel to the Albany Hotel in Glasgow for an interview with me. Not only did he accommodate me with a change in schedule, but he actually brought along his own tape recorder, since by this time mine was broken.

Dr. Campbell is a fifty-six-year-old longtime comrade of Mr. Cameron's. He has the usual ruddy Scottish complexion. I found him as forthright, positive, and conservative as his Scottish accent. When he first arrived we chatted about his hobbies: golf and amateur radio. He contacts New Zealand almost every morning. That day he had spoken to someone in Little Rock, Arkansas.

Dr. Campbell is a consultant physician for Lanarkshire Hospitals and works out of Hairmyres Hospital in East Kilbride, Scotland.

INTERVIEW WITH DR. ALLAN CAMPBELL

H. L. NEWBOLD: Dr. Campbell, how did you get interested in using vitamin C to treat cancer patients?

39

A. CAMPBELL: When Ewan Cameron and I worked in the hospital together many years ago we were interested in various aspects of cancer. When Cameron started applying his basic theories about the use of ascorbic acid to help people with cancer, he asked me to help with the clinical work.

HLN: That was in 1971, or when?

AC: I think it was 1973 or thereabouts when I took on my present hospital appointment and we started our cooperative research. We had been friends and colleagues for many years. Our paths and interests have diverged over the years. I have been interested in other things, but still keep going back again into the study of ascorbic acid.

HLN: Do you use the same dosage he uses when you treat patients?

AC: Yes, I think the doses we use are quite similar, but at the present time I have a patient on 50 grams a day. This is a very special patient who comes into the hospital periodically for intravenous doses of 20 to 30 grams a day, but, generally speaking, she takes from 10 to 30 grams a day by mouth.

HLN: You administer it intravenously?

AC: In hospital part is given intravenous and part by mouth, usually somewhere around 20 grams a day intravenously by continuous infusion and 30 grams by mouth, but the dosage varies.

HLN: What is special about the patient you mentioned?

AC: This woman has a leiomyosarcoma, confirmed by biopsy, which was treated some years ago with chemotherapy. I was asked to see this lady specifically because she had so much abdominal pain that she had become addicted to heroin and her general physician asked if I knew anything that could be done about this. At that time she was very emaciated and very unwell and she had a very distended abdomen with large masses of tumor. We took her into the hospital, and after about three weeks of treatment with ascorbic acid everything quieted down. She put on about a stone [fourteen pounds] of weight. She felt quite better,

40

and her hair, which had fallen out because of the chemotherapy, gradually grew in. She is not cured of cancer by any means, but she has now had approximately three relatively good years.

It is interesting that on occasions when she has stopped the treatment for some reason, within forty-eight hours the tumor has flared up and she has had to be sent to the hospital again. I'm afraid we are reaching some sort of end point with this remarkable woman. She comes in with severe abdominal pain. Her abdomen is extended with tumor masses. Now, at this stage, the tumors no longer shrink after we give her ascorbic acid, but the abdomen becomes much softer. She spends her time walking about the hospital with her intravenous infusion hanging over her shoulder. She has been going through this for about three years. I think she has greatly benefited from the treatment. Let me make it quite clear, however, and I think Mr. Cameron would agree, that we're very Scottish and not a little careful. We're almost doubting Thomases. I think it is very dangerous to get carried away with excessive enthusiasm, but I think undoubtedly everybody who has observed this lady feels she is deriving benefit from the treatment and it's not just care in the hospital and it's not just hydration that has helped her, because it takes up to three weeks before she experiences considerable remission of symptoms and the distension of her abdomen goes down. She is obviously deriving benefit from the ascorbic acid.

HLN: She's how old?

AC: She's in her thirties.

HLN: Is she a housewife?

AC: She is a housewife. This treatment with ascorbic acid, incidentally, has been in addition to prednisone [an adrenal cortical hormone] treatment. She has been on prednisone continuously since the chemotherapy treatments, so we are simply adding ascorbic acid.

HLN: Are you using chemotherapy simultaneously with ascorbic acid?

AC: I don't often, because in this country we've got

oncologists who do most of the chemotherapy. But from time to time we get cases referred from them. This particular girl, for example, has been followed passively by the oncologist. He feels she does not need other treatment because she is doing well with the ascorbic acid.

HLN: When will they refer chemotherapy patients to you?

AC: Unfortunately, most of them are referred only when things are pretty grim. I think this is proper until we finally determine the efficacy of the ascorbic acid by properly controlled trials. I think it is fair to first try the proven and accepted forms of treatment, within reason.

HLN: Have chemotherapy studies been done on cancer with controls?

AC: I think quite a lot of work has been done on this. The reports vary, of course. I was recently at a conference on the treatment of lymphomas. Stages 1 and 2 lymphomas do very well on chemotherapy, but stages 3 and 4 do just as well without chemotherapy. It is a very difficult subject to assess.

HLN: Has the chemotherapist done controls like yours and Cameron's?

AC: That I don't know. I shouldn't think so. It is a very difficult thing to do controlled experiments on people with cancer. The patients we treat are often terminally ill, so it's a different kettle of fish. It is ethical for us to use controls.

HLN: In a way this makes your work more scientific than the work done with chemotherapy.

AC: Perhaps so.

HLN: Do some patients get chemotherapy and ascorbic acid together?

AC: Yes, we've treated one or two that way. There has been a gradual acceptance of the possibility of using the two together. In my own particular experience I am just at the beginning of this co-operation and acceptance. I think you've got to move slowly, you've got to make your points with your colleagues.

HLN: Then there is no contraindication for using them together?

AC: The only possible contraindication might be that if ascorbic acid is a very good detoxifying agent then it might possibly detoxify the chemotherapy and annul or relatively annul the effect on the cancer cells.

HLN: How are you going to find out?

AC: That's a difficult problem. I'm not sure. That's one thing we've got to think about.

HLN: What do the oncologists say about this problem?

AC: I haven't discussed this point with them. These ideas are just beginning to evolve. We've had patients who can apparently tolerate maximum chemotherapy much better when they are also on ascorbic acid. I haven't personally used this approach, but Mr. Cameron has told me about it. It may be that patients are tolerating larger amounts of the chemotherapy simply because the chemical is detoxified by the ascorbic acid.

I met some Japanese physicians who first administer chemotherapy and then give large doses of the ascorbic acid after the chemotherapy. This tended to annul the toxic side effects of the chemotherapy.

HLN: What would you do if you had cancer?

AC: I think that if I had cancer, or if any of my family had cancer, I would undergo reasonable amounts of the standard forms of therapy.

I would like to stress that I think it vitally important that the patient be prepared for the onslaught of cancer treatment with proper nutrition, including large amounts of vitamin C. Often somebody who has suffered for a considerable period of time from a malignant tumor is in poor shape and must be revitalized with proper nutrition. Such a patient will be undergoing a very stressful treatment following immediately upon the stress of surgery. To jump in and give X-ray treatment and chemotherapy without paying special attention to the patients' nutritional needs is very bad. I have a feeling that physicians, all of us, should be thinking about this matter of nutrition more than we do. The stronger the patients are, the greater chance we have to save them. We must be very careful not to destroy the natural defense mechanisms of the body.

We must preserve as much of the body's natural defense mechanisms as possible. Ascorbic acid in massive doses is a great help in this matter.

HLN: And good nutrition helps in resistance.

AC: I am sure that is true. I think you read the paper on the single case we had of reticular cell sarcoma we treated.

HLN: The patient who went into remission and then relapsed?

AC: This was a patient of mine, really. At the time, though, three of us were involved. In this case, the ascorbic acid acted almost as if it were a chemotherapeutic agent.

HLN: I think our readers would like to know more about this patient. Can you give us some details?

AC: He was a lorryman, who you call in the States a truck driver. He presented a three-month history of being vaguely unwell, and towards the end of this three months he developed enlarged glands in his neck, a large liver, and an enlarged spleen, was running a temperature, had lost weight and appetite, and was just generally a very unwell man.

HLN: He was how old?

AC: He was forty-two at that time.

The glands in his neck were so big that the resident physicians were taken to the end of the ward and asked to look at the patient and make a diagnosis. All of them said it looked like Hodgkin's disease and/or a malignant lymphoma. Unfortunately, we didn't take a picture of this chap, but the glands were obvious and a biopsy suggested a reticulum cell sarcoma. We arranged for the oncologist to take him over for therapy. There was a delay of ten days for him to get a bed at the hospital where the oncologist practiced. This delay prompted me to put the patient on ascorbic acid over the weekend just to see what would happen. I began his treatment on Friday. He was given 10 grams of ascorbic acid intravenously daily.

When I came in to see him on Tuesday, the glands in his neck had almost disappeared. His fever had gone. By the end of three weeks all of the obvious signs of illness had vanished. An X ray of the chest was now normal. He was eating well and feeling well. Then he was put on oral therapy—10 grams of ascorbic acid daily. This was October.

By January we thought we could start reducing his ascorbic acid. By March we had stopped the treatment.

About a month later, however, he wasn't feeling so well. He was losing weight, had a bit of a cough, and his chest X ray showed a return of the enlarged glands in the mediastinum. He returned to the hospital, where he began his ascorbic acid therapy again. We gave him 20 grams a day, part oral and part intravenous. He has now been well for four years and takes 12.5 grams of ascorbic acid per day. He's back at work full time.

Later he developed a small nodule in his thyroid gland. The surgeon who removed it reported it as a cyst. But further examination showed it to be a low-grade carcinoma of the thyroid. This was an extremely interesting development, because this developed while he was on large doses of ascorbic acid. The general opinion was that the thyroid should be operated. He tolerated the surgery very well, and there is no evidence of his reticulum cell sarcoma.

So here's a case of reticulum cell sarcoma with metastasis [spreading] that was completely controlled by the use of ascorbic acid.

One might argue that the first remission was spontaneous remission, but the fact that he relapsed when the ascorbic acid was stopped and then remitted again when the ascorbic acid was restarted cancels out that argument.

HLN: Do you think ascorbic acid is more effective if given by vein?

AC: I don't really think so. It gets the patient started, but when the patient is better you can switch over to giving it by mouth.

HLN: Why don't you use larger amounts of ascorbic acid by mouth?

AC: Well, I have used larger amounts. I have used

45

up to 30 grams a day by mouth. But many of my patients find the larger doses upset them a little.

To get back to the truck driver—the trouble is that one doesn't often come across a situation like the truck driver, because they tend to go into conventional ways of treatment. This was just a fluke. I think this was a good fluke, because it saved the man a lot of trauma. It saved him from chemotherapy. Yet, if later he should need chemotherapy, it's there waiting for him. He hasn't exhausted his chemotherapy. This is all to the good. I would imagine that if he had had the chemotherapy before the ascorbic acid and then relapsed, the ascorbic acid might not have been so effective.

HLN: Again, what exactly would you do if you had cancer?

AC: I would have surgery if possible. It would depend. Chemotherapy and X-ray therapy would have to be very carefully considered before I would have it. I would need to be certain in my own mind that the treatment was not going to be worse than the disease.

HLN: As Dr. Charles Huggins says, some things are worse than death.

AC: Yes, I think that is true. But we've got to appreciate the situation of the doctor in this case. He is faced with a desperate situation, and desperate diseases sometimes require desperate treatment.

HLN: Chemotherapy can certainly ruin the quality of a patient's last months of life.

AC: This is true, and therefore one has got to realize that the last months of life have got to pay dividends. Unfortunately, in many cases where chemotherapy is used it doesn't. You've got to take into account each individual case.

HLN: So you might or might not take chemotherapy and X-ray treatment. Would you perhaps take a trial for a few weeks on ascorbic acid and then evaluate the results?

AC: I suppose I might. I think it would be very difficult to decide. I would have to ask for the help of my colleagues to make a decision about myself. I think that the decision in the late stage of disease would be easier to make than in the early stages, but in the early stages you would have to seek specialized guidance.

HLN: If you decided to take chemotherapy, would you take ascorbic acid with it?

AC: If I were pressed on that point, I think I would probably do so.

HLN: Perhaps in a hundred years there may be many more-definite answers, but that won't help us now. Do you take vitamin C yourself?

AC: From time to time. I took it for approximately two or three years, about 1 gram a day, and then I stopped it. But I take it from time to time. Today I took about 4 grams, because I felt I had a cold coming on.

HLN: Of course, upper respiratory infection is one of the things that does cancer patients in rather frequently.

AC: Well, I think that is true. Any devitalizing disease like cancer will increase a patient's susceptibility to infections. So if ascorbic acid does increase the resistance to these infections, that is all to the good. Even if it did not help destroy the cancer, it might help ward off infections. I think the total nutrition of the patient is also important.

HLN: What do you think about vitamin C as a preventive for cancer?

AC: I find that this is not a viable proposition. If it is correct that many members of the animal kingdom manufacture 2 to 4 grams of ascorbic acid a day, it certainly doesn't give them immunity from neoplasms [tumors]. So I don't think this is a viable proposition.

HLN: But it is true that everyone is exposed to things that cause cancer, such as viruses and chemicals, but only some people get it.

AC: I think this is true, but there are other factors. There are genetic factors.

HLN: What form of vitamin C do you use the most by mouth?

AC: We give what is called a Vale of Leven mixture—a mixture of sodium ascorbate, sodium bicarbonate, ascorbic acid, and sorbitol.

HLN: Do you use a fine ascorbic acid powder or the coarse powder?

AC: You've asked me a question which I'm not certain about, but I think I've seen them making it up with a fine powder.

HLN: Do you use calcium ascorbate?

AC: I've seen it used.

HLN: Do you recommend other vitamins or any diet for cancer patients?

AC: No.

HLN: If patient resistance is part of the problem, why don't you add more vitamins and minerals to the diet?

AC: That is certainly a good question. I think we try to give these people as good and balanced a diet as possible, but we personally have only been interested in the effect of ascorbic acid. There is evidence that vitamin E may have some effect on cancer. This is possibly true.

HLN: What you are thinking about is your research protocol?

AC: What we're trying to really determine is if the addition of ascorbic acid to conventional treatments for cancer is going to add to the survival rates of these patients.

HLN: If you had cancer, would you take other vitamins in addition to vitamin C?

AC: Possibly I would. We tend to give supplemental vitamins of the B group on the ward, but not in large amounts.

I think we have reasonable evidence that ascorbic acid helps almost certainly in some cases.

I'm convinced that in individual cases you can improve the quality of life . . . patients feel better, have an elevated mood and less pain.

HLN: This is true for the general population, too, when they take ascorbic acid in large amounts.

AC: I'm sure this is true. Many people with mental diseases also feel better on quite a lot of ascorbic acid. So even on the basis of making cancer patients feel better during the last months of life, vitamin C is very helpful. Anything that improves the quality of life, the subjective quality of life, is important.

We have a lady, a patient of my colleague Dr. Jack, who presented herself to the doctor a few years ago with rheumatoid arthritis and enlarged glands and spleen. Even with a biopsy there was some doubt about the diagnosis. She was put on ascorbic acid, and her glands disappeared and everything settled down. She was kept on ascorbic acid for some time—two or three years, I think. Then it was stopped, and, regrettably, she relapsed very quickly. A second biopsy of a gland showed very clearly that this was a malignant lymphoma. This time she went downhill very rapidly in spite of vitamin C. Now it may well be that the original remission was due to the ascorbic acid, if we take the truck driver as an example. And it might well be that if the ascorbic acid had not been stopped she might not have relapsed.

HLN: What are your views on Laetrile?

AC: On my way to New Zealand a few years ago, I stopped in California and met some very nice people there who were very hospitable, but I didn't get answers that satisfied my Scottish nature. It may be that Laetrile fits in, but I don't know of any scientific claims that support it.

HLN: Some people would like to put vitamin C in the same category as Laetrile, but the quality of work that has been done with vitamin C is very different. You have used proper controls.

AC: We have been very careful, and I think you will agree that ascorbic acid has been of benefit to many cancer patients. Its full usefulness is still to be defined.

HLN: This woman that you spoke of, how old was she? Was she a housewife? What did she have to say about the usefulness of ascorbic acid?

AC: She was in her fifties, I believe, a housewife. I think she was very pleased with the results ascorbic acid gave her.

49

HLN: I understand that patients in Scotland are often not told they have cancer.

AC: Well, we don't broadcast it. If a patient asks specifically, yes, we tell him. I think that's fair, but I personally don't think you should tell a patient unless he asks.

HLN: If a patient goes to surgery and comes back, doesn't he want to know what was found?

AC: Yes, that is true. We try to be as honest as possible, but we try to limit the information given them. I think that is kindness and reasonableness. Patients who are going to die from cancer know soon enough.

HLN: What do you think is the most important thing to tell people about ascorbic acid and cancer?

AC: I'm sure that the one thing they should not be told is that vitamin C is a cure for cancer. I do not think that false hopes should be built up about this. My own feelings, and I think Ewan Cameron agrees, are that ascorbic acid often greatly improves the quality of life of the cancer patient and helps him live longer. Whether or not it is a curative in some cases we still don't know. I think Cameron would agree with me that vitamin C's exact position in the therapy of cancer is still to be defined. I think before you convince the medical world you've got to have properly organized control trials. I have a feeling that the trial which was designed by Ewan Cameron using terminally ill cancer patients was the best approach. Generally speaking, I don't think vitamin C should be used alone to treat cancer. There may be exceptions, of course. There may be a patient who cannot take other treatment because of physical or mental illness.

6

Discoverer of Vitamin C: Albert Szent-Györgyi

In 1937 a Nobel prize was awarded to Hungarian-born Albert Szent-Györgyi for isolating chemically pure vitamin C.

The scientist had observed that certain fruits contained a substance that seemed to have a protective effect against disease. His first name for the unknown substance was *ignose,* because he was completely ignorant of what it might be. He later referred to it as *God-knows,* because only God knew what it was.

Today we know the substance as vitamin C.

His first supplies came from the adrenal glands of cattle. It took him a whole year to collect 15 grams (about 4 teaspoons).

While at the University of Szeged, in Hungary's paprika-growing region, he decided that paprika might be a rich source of *God-knows.* Within a month he had prepared more than 3 pounds of the treasured white powder.

I've known Albert Szent-Györgyi for years, have been on the speaker's platform with him, and have had a chance to talk with him several times. The last time I saw him was in the spring of 1978, at a medical meeting in Palm Springs called to celebrate the fiftieth anniversary of his discovery.

Szent-Györgyi is in his mid-eighties, but he still has a sparkle in his eye and is not above making a ribald joke at the beginning of one of his scientific presentations.

Interview with Dr. Albert Szent-Györgyi

H. L. Newbold: Number one: Do you think vitamin C is important in the treatment and prevention of cancer?

A. Szent-Györgyi: Well, this whole problem is now in development. It's very complicated. But vitamin C seems to be very important. Very much important.

HLN: Do you think it is very important in both prevention and treatment?

AS-G: Yes, it's very much involved.

HLN: And what do you think the mechanism is for it?

AS-G: Oh, you ask something! I worked twenty years to find this out. It's very complicated. It's a very complex chemical mechanism. It cannot be explained in a few words.

HLN: Everything can be explained in a few words.

AS-G: No, no, I can't.

HLN: You talk about electronic acceptors, about vitamin C, ascorbic acid, being an electronic acceptor. What does this have to do with cancer? . . .

AS-G: All living phenomena are to a great extent electronic phenomena. And cancer is also an electron disease. Because all really complex living reactions are electronic reactions, not molecular.

HLN: And do you feel that cancer is a defect in electron transfer?

AS-G: Yes.

HLN: And you think because vitamin C facilitates this transfer, that's why it's applicable?

AS-G: Yes. Vitamin C is involved in electron transfers.

HLN: And you think that's why it's useful for cancer treatment?

AS-G: Yes.

HLN: Do you have any idea about the dosage the average person should take in the prevention of cancer?

AS-G: Oh, no, I couldn't say anything about that. I'm a theoretical chemist myself.

HLN: Yes, I know. But you must have some thoughts about it.

AS-G: I have only personal experience. But I wouldn't like to act as an authority on medication.

HLN: What if you had cancer, what would you do?

AS-G: Well, I would take ascorbic acid, and I don't know what else I would do. . . . It is a problem what I would do. I don't know enough about the treatment of cancer.

HLN: Would you take massive amounts of vitamin C?

AS-G: Vitamin C I would take, certainly.

HLN: How much would you take?

AS-G: Well, I don't know. I would take 5 grams a day or something like that. The people who work on cancer, like Dr. Cameron in Scotland—he gives 10 grams a day.

HLN: What do you think of the work that's been done by Dr. Cameron? Have you read his paper?

AS-G: Oh yes, yes, certainly.

HLN: What is your evaluation of that work?

AS-G: It's very good work. I visited Dr. Cameron. He's a very fine fellow.

HLN: Do you find him and his work scientifically sound?

AS-G: Yes, definitely.

HLN: Do you have any criticism of the way the paper is put together?

AS-G: No, no. It's all very good work he does.

HLN: What do you think the general public should know regarding vitamin C and cancer?

AS-G: Well, that there is some connection between vitamin C and cancer and what Cameron has published is all right.

HLN: You would follow Cameron's advice?

AS-G: Yes.

HLN: Anything else you'd like to tell me . . . ?
AS-G: No . . . only that we are working very hard.

Szent-Györgyi's life reads like a novel. Through it weave royal families and escapes from conquering armies. Tossed here and there by fate, he has at last found a true home in one of the most improbable places on earth: Woods Hole, a picturesque old whaling village on Cape Cod.

In 1973, Tamara and Franklin Salisbury of Bethesda, Maryland, happened to see a newspaper story about a Nobel prize-winning scientist named Albert Szent-Györgyi who could not get government funds to carry on his cancer research. After sending him a twenty-five dollar donation, they were amazed to get a charming letter of thanks.

They soon met the scientist, and were so impressed that they decided to form a nonprofit corporation to help him, the National Foundation for Cancer Research. Today they have 350,000 members and have raised two and a half million dollars, mostly in tens and twenties from the average Joe in the street who wanted to do something to help fight cancer. Anyone wishing to help can send a tax-deductible donation to the National Foundation for Cancer Research in Bethesda, Maryland.

Today Dr. Szent-Györgyi does cancer research full time. Since he lost both his wife and only child to cancer, he has a personal stake in his work.

Little by little he feels he is beginning to understand the molecular causes of cancer.

Here—in an article he wrote for *Executive Health,* May 1978—is what he has to say on the subject.

How New Understandings about the Biological Function of Ascorbic Acid May Profoundly Affect Our Lives
By Albert Szent-Györgyi

In a remarkably short time after we discovered ascorbic acid fifty years ago, we knew everything about its structure that was worth knowing . . . but its biological function remained unknown. It was not possible to use it intelligently as long as we did not know how it functioned. "We can control only what we understand." Without such an understanding we could not decide even simple questions. Take, for example, the long controversy over the so-called "Minimum Daily Requirements" (MDR) . . . because no one knew for sure how ascorbic acid functioned in our bodies. Now my associates and I have found out how and this new understanding opens vast new vistas for its use in medicine. But let us begin at the beginning.

We divide the surrounding world into animate and inanimate, that is alive and not alive. The division is sharp, unequivocal. It is very rarely that we are in doubt where something belongs. What characterizes life is its wonderful, subtle reactivity. There has to be some fundamental difference between the living and the lifeless. The definition of this difference in terms of exact sciences is one of the main problems of biology on which the solution to many important medical problems depends.

The main bearer of life is protein, so one expects that proteins share with living systems their reactivity. They do not! Apart from enzymic activity, they show no special reactivity at all. Proteins are built of relatively clumsy large molecules (macromolecules) in which the electrons, the small electric particles which surround the atomic nuclei (core), are held firmly in their places and have no mobility.

Approaching this problem four decades ago I felt that the wonderful reactivity of the living cell cannot be generated by unreactive, clumsily large molecules and the real actors of life had to be much smaller and more mobile.

They could hardly be anything else than electrons.* The proteins consisting of large molecules could not be the actors. They had to be, rather, the stage on which the drama of life was enacted. To be mobile, electrons need a conductor which made me propose (1941) that proteins may be conductors. My proposition was unanimously rejected for the simple reason that none of the great number of proteins which were isolated and thoroughly studied showed any signs of semiconductivity. Biology was and is a molecular science which took little cognizance of the electronic dimension.

The only way in which I could explain this situation to myself was by supposing that the same protein which showed no signs of life in vitro was in a different physico-chemical state in vivo, in the living cell. I called this physico-chemical state in which I supposed the proteins to be in the living system "the living state."

To avoid misunderstanding and confusion I must interject here that there is no such thing as "the protein." Proteins are exceedingly versatile substances which, in the living organism, perform very different functions, some of which are very simple and demand no special reactivity and conductivity, and so what I will say pertains only to the proteins which partake in the generation of the great signs of life, like motion, secretion, excitability.

This difference between the live proteins within the living organism and the same proteins after they have been purified and isolated presents in a nutshell the difference between the animate and inanimate world, and my problem boiled down to defining this difference.

The first question which had to be answered was this: is there a method by which an unreactive protein macromolecule can be transformed into a highly reactive one? There is one way, and this is by taking out single electrons from it. In the protein molecule the electrons form pairs, the two electrons of the pair spinning in opposite directions. A spinning electron is a little magnet, and the two electrons of the pair represent opposed charged magnets

---

* Electrons are elementary particles that are a fundamental constituent of matter, having a negative charge, a mass, a spin, and are components of an atom outside the nucleus.

compensating each other's magnetic moments, which strongly couples them. Taking out single electrons from a molecule requires that electron pairs have to be separated, uncoupled. A molecule containing an uncoupled electron is called a "free radical" and free radicals are known to be highly reactive. They contain not only an uncoupled electron, they contain also half-filled orbitals, the eliminated electron leaving a positively charged "electron hole" behind. All this upsets the balance of the molecule and makes it highly reactive.

The protein molecule has only a definite number of places (orbitals) on which it can hold electrons. If all these places are occupied by electrons then there can be no electronic mobility. The situation is similar to a completely filled parking lot. To induce mobility a car has to be taken out. This makes all the rest mobile. So my problem was: how can electrons be taken out of a protein molecule?

Electrons can be taken out of a protein molecule by "electron acceptors," that is, other molecules which have an empty orbital on which they can accommodate an additional electron. The transfer of single electrons from a "donor" to an "acceptor" is called "charge transfer," which is one of the most important biological reactions. The electron transferred from the donor to the acceptor will oscillate between the two. What part of its time it will spend on the acceptors depends on energy relations. If it spends only a small part of its time there, then it is customary to say that only "a small part of the electron" has been transferred—the half, one tenth, a hundredth, as the case may be.

The situation in most organic molecules, as well as in proteins, is similar to the situation in a completely filled parking lot in which (as I said) no single place is free, in which all cars are immobile. By taking out one car all the cars become mobilized, there being one free place now which allows shuffling. So in proteins too, taking out one (or more) electrons makes all the electrons mobile. To have the electrons mobile the protein must be desaturated electronically. The more it is desaturated, the more electrons are taken out, the more mobile the other electrons will be.

All this, taken together, opens the possibility that the basic difference between "alive" and "not alive" is an electronic desaturation. While in inanimate systems the molecules are "closed shell molecules" in which all allowed places (orbitals) are occupied by electron pairs, in living systems the proteins are desaturated electronically, the living state of protein being the desaturated, free radical state. Desaturation depends on the availability of electron acceptors which can take the electrons out of the proteins.*

When the number of unpaired electrons formed is small it means that only a small part of the electrons has gone over and the charge transfer is a weak one. Such a weak charge transfer can lead only to a low degree of desaturation of protein. This is very important because when life originated billions of years ago, our globe was covered by dense water vapor, and there was no light and no oxygen at the surface, and the only acceptor available was methylglyoxal (MG) that could produce only a low level of protein desaturation. So, in this first dark and anaerobic

---

* The research of my laboratory showed that the main acceptor used by animal cells is methylglyoxal (MG).

It was discovered more than sixty years ago that all living systems studied contained a most active enzyme, a "glyoxalase," for the inactivation of methylglyoxal (its conversion into D-lactic acid). Actually glyoxalase is two enzymes, glyoxalase I and II which use SH-glutathione as coenzyme. Nature does not indulge in luxuries, and if there is such a highly active ubiquitous enzymic system, it must have something very important to do, but nobody could find out what. A role in the desaturation of protein would fully justify its existence.

MG can attack proteins by interacting with its aldehydic group, with the 2 NH_2 (amino) groups of protein. The reaction between $C = 0$ and NH_2 being possibly one of the most central reactions of cell life demands a more thorough study. Proteins being very complex, I started this study with simple models containing methylamine, MA, instead of protein, MA being the simplest aliphatic amine.

Mixing a watery solution of MA and MG a dark color develops, indicating that reaction occurred. As shown by Gascoyne, in the ESR spectroscope the solution gave a strong signal, which meant that electrons have gone over from MA to MG. Charge transfer occurred.

(oxygen-free) period of life only the simplest, most primitive living forms were developed.

This situation changed when, owing to cooling, the water vapor envelope of our globe condensed and, eventually, light could reach the surface of the globe. Life captured the photons of this light and used their energy for separating the elements of water (H and O), producing free oxygen, which is a very strong electron acceptor. This opened the way to development and differentiation . . . the end result today is us!

I have called the first dark and anerobic period of life the α period. In this period only the simple organisms could be built which could perform only the simplest reactions, the most important of which was proliferation, which was favored by the simplicity of structure and made life perennial. The subsequent anaerobic and light period I called the β period. In it life developed increasingly complex structures capable of increasingly complex and subtle reactions, while proliferation was subjected to regulation. In this β period proliferation must have been inhibited by the solid structures built and strong cohesive forces developed to hold these structures together. The cohesive forces, as shown by Laki and Ladik, were greatly enforced by the electronic desaturation of protein.

What lends an acute interest to these reactions is the fact that they are not limited to the far distant past. Structures and cohesion interfere with cell division, so a dividing cell has to disassemble its structures and relax its cohesive forces; it has to return to an extent to the α state.

The $\alpha \leftarrow \rightarrow \beta$ transformation had thus to be reversible and occur in every cell division. All dividing cells have to be in the α state which explains why all dividing cells (embryonic and cancer cells alike) have very similar properties. After cell division is completed the cell has to build up its β state again. Should this state become unstable, then the cell has to persist in the proliferative α state, and tumor results!

The next question we had to answer was: how did oxygen desaturate the protein? If free oxygen would attack protein we would burn up!

Here is where ascorbic acid assumes a basic role in the

59

mechanisms of life. It is present in tissues as a salt, ascorbate. As Gascoyne has found, when ascorbate meets oxygen it passes onto it one of its electrons, and becomes itself a very reactive free radical. This radical, having lost an electron. is a very good electron acceptor which can readily take a whole electron from the methylglyoxal, attached to the protein. This means that the protein becomes desaturated, becomes a reactive conductant free radical. Its electron is passed to methylglyoxal, methylglyoxal passes it on to ascorbate (which has made room for it by giving an electron to oxygen). The real final electron acceptor of protein is thus the oxygen.

In this process in which the protein is transduced into the living state, ascorbic acid plays a central role. Without it no electrons can be transmitted to oxygen and the protein cannot be desaturated.

McLaughlin discovered that these charge transfer reactions lead to the production of free radicals which can be studied in the light spectroscope. In the interaction of methylglyoxal, methylamine and ascorbic acid and oxygen two free radicals are formed, one with a maximum of absorption at 380 and another with a maximum of absorptions around 475 nm.* Pethig, Bone, Lewis, and myself have shown that if protein is treated with methylglyoxal it turns brown, assuming the color of liver, and becomes an electronic conductor. (This explained why the liver is brown.) Methylglyoxal can actually be isolated from the liver proteins.

Does all this help us to decide how to apply ascorbic acid? It does! It also explains the difference between ascorbic acid and other vitamins. Other vitamins have a favorable action on health only as they correct a deficiency, be it small or great!

Ascorbic acid, transducing the protein into the living state, enables it to perform. The more ascorbic acid is available, the better the protein will work.

The spectroscopic observations (mentioned above) indicate that methylglyoxal and ascorbic acid are incorporated into the protein, linked to it by covalent bonds. The

---

* Nanometers. One nanometer equals a billionth of a meter.—HLN

protein is thus activated by incorporating into it the acceptor.

The ascorbic acid ingested by man is excreted only partly with his urine. Its greatest part simply disappears! What happened to it was a mystery. My studies indicate that it is incorporated into the living machinery!

This brings out a point which is important in relation to medical application. To have a well functioning cellular machinery the ascorbic acid must be available while the machine is built.

(If we build a wall, the mortar must be applied to every brick. One does not raise a wall putting bricks together and then pouring cement over them.) So one should not wait for the application of this vitamin until one gets ill, trying to put the situation right by taking big doses. We should take it all the time.

To have plenty of ascorbic acid is especially important in our young years when we build our body. But ascorbic acid should be available at all ages. The older we become the less we are able to store and use it, thus the more we need of it.

(No doubt, we can stay alive on very small doses, as a car can run also without servicing. The difference will only be that without good servicing the car will become useless after 50,000 miles, while with good service it may last several times as long.)

The electronic desaturation of protein greatly increases the cohesive force holding the living structures together. This explains why in scurvy old scars open up. In absence of ascorbic acid the cohesive forces weaken. Ascorbic acid is needed to keep these cohesive forces at a maximum which prevents the body falling apart.

The action of ascorbic acid on cohesion leads also to another important conclusion about the ascorbic acid medication. We need ascorbic acid not only for holding our body together, but also for putting it together. Without sufficient ascorbic acid the body cells cannot be built precisely. This is very important because if a body has been left without a satisfactory ascorbic acid supply for a long period, the damage cannot be put right by a big dose of ascorbic acid.

As you know, a full grown human of 60 kg needs about

60 grams of protein daily in his food to stay in nutritional balance. This means that 60 grams of protein have to be remade daily. Without sufficient ascorbic acid the cells cannot be put together correctly, and if they were put together in an unsatisfactory manner it has to take a long time to put the damage straight. In my calculations it takes six months to put such damage right, six months during which the body has been supplied with ample ascorbic acid, at least 2–8 grams daily.

Last year I collected a rather unfortunate personal experience on this. I broke down with pneumonia which I could not shake off for months, until I discovered that the quantities of ascorbic acid which I took (1 gram daily) had become insufficient at my age (84). When I went up from 1 gram to eight, my troubles were over.

I strongly believe that a proper use of ascorbic acid can profoundly change our vital statistics, including those for cancer. For this, ascorbic acid would have to cease to be looked upon as a medicine, sold in milligram pills by the druggist. It would have to become a household article, like sugar and salt and flour, sold in the supermarket in powder form by the pound.

Ascorbic acid is a vitamin which has to be taken as a food because mankind grew up in the tropical jungle where there was plenty of it and there was no need to make it. I suspect that the lost paradise of the old biblical story was actually the tropical jungle with its ample supply of ascorbic acid.

During my long research career I have become deeply impressed by the perfection of the human body. All those diseases, about which I had to learn as a medical student, are to a great extent due to our abuse, our mishandling of our body, in which a lack of ascorbate plays an important role. Present medicine is lopsided. As a medical student I had to listen no end to lectures on disease, but cannot remember one on health, full health!

7

William Saccoman

It isn't often the general public gets to listen in on a
private conversation between two physicians. In this
chapter, however, you have a chance to read a tran-
script from the uncensored taped interview I had with
Dr. William J. Saccoman, of San Diego, California.

You must forgive some repetition of material from
other chapters. Each man I talked with held some
views in common with others, but each also had some
special contribution of his own. In order to get the
full rounded picture we need every view.

Conversations such as you are about to read take
place all over the world between doctors who are
using new techniques and working on new discoveries.
Dr. Joseph Burchenal, director of clinical investigation at Memorial Hospital for Cancer and Allied
Diseases, for example, says that he makes it a point to
stay on a first-name basis with fellow physicians in his
field all around the world—from Moscow to Western
Europe to Japan.

INTERVIEW WITH DR. SACCOMAN

H. L. NEWBOLD: Dr. Saccoman, this is Dr. Newbold
in New York. Irwin Stone gave me your name. I am a
physician writing a book on vitamin C and cancer.
I'd like to ask some questions about your experiences
and techniques, and perhaps get some advice.

W. SACCOMAN: Well, I've been using vitamin C to

treat cancer patients since 1971. It has been very gratifying in a good many instances. I've also had some very profound disappointments, mostly with patients who had chemotherapy before seeing me.

HLN: How do you mean?

WS: Some of the patients who had chemotherapy before getting vitamin C just didn't seem to respond.

HLN: They had chemotherapy first? Or concurrently?

WS: First. I have a few patients that have used chemotherapy and the vitamin C together, and that has been very gratifying.

HLN: That's worked out well, has it?

WS: Yes, the vitamin C apparently helps protect the healthy body cells against the toxicity of the chemotherapeutic agent.

HLN: Since vitamin C is such a strong detoxifier, the question has come up whether the vitamin will protect the cancer cells as well as the healthy cells.

WS: That is something I have wondered about also.

HLN: And what's your conclusion?

WS: I don't believe the vitamin C keeps the chemotherapeutic agents from attacking the cancerous cells.

HLN: It's very interesting to hear about your experience. Have you had very many patients with the combination of chemotherapy and vitamin C?

WS: I've had five of them, and all of them are still living.

HLN: Very interesting.

WS: One with a grade 4 lymphosarcoma.

HLN: And these were biopsy-proven?

WS: Yes.

HLN: Have you treated any skin cancer?

WS: Not with vitamin C alone. Most of the skin cancer has had surgical removal.

HLN: What dosage of vitamin C have you used to treat cancer?

WS: Well, I started out very cautiously and gradually worked up. The dosage that seems most effective is 1 gram per kilogram [2.2 pounds] per day, preferably spread out through the entire day.

HLN: Which form do you use?

WS: I've been using powdered sodium ascorbate mixed with powdered ascorbic acid during the daytime, and prolonged-acting ascorbic acid tablets at night. Usually I start them out with intravenous infusions right here in the office.

HLN: What dosage?

WS: Thirty grams I.V. in 500 cc's of Ringer's lactate over a period of about three hours.

HLN: Do you add any calcium to that?

WS: No, I haven't had any tetany [neuromuscular hyperactivity] or anything like that.

HLN: How many days do you give it intravenously?

WS: Usually I give it intravenously until the patient can take it by mouth. That takes ten days to three weeks. I also give them advice on nutrition . . .

HLN: If they can take it by mouth straight away, do you start it by mouth?

WS: Yes.

HLN: These are only people who are quite ill that you . . .

WS: Yes, I start it by vein only in patients who are terminally ill. They're in terrible shape nutritionally.

I want you to understand, Dr. Newbold, that I don't think vitamin C is a cure for cancer, but I certainly think it's a super adjunctive treatment.

HLN: You think it prolongs life in cancer patients and makes the quality of life better?

WS: Yes, this is exactly it. It gives the patient a marvelous immediate sense of well-being after one infusion. What experience do you have with it?

HLN: I got started with a patient, a fifty-six-year-old woman, with an oat cell carcinoma of the lung discovered last May. She was on chemotherapy until November of last year and got so sick that she just refused to take any more. She came to see me and wanted to know what I had to offer her. I started her on ascorbic acid on December 13. She improved a great deal. She was nauseated when she first saw me. I started her off with 5 grams intravenously twice a day for three or four days and then gradually got her onto oral ascorbic acid. Now she's on 48 grams a day, and has been for some time. She's felt very good right away and has done very well. At Memorial Hospital they said she'd be back at the end of December begging for more chemotherapy. They've been surprised how well she's done, but she went back the other day * and got a chest X ray and they found a quarter-size return in her lung. She doesn't want any more chemotherapy. I wanted to get your advice about what to do, whether I should increase her vitamin C or try to get her to take the chemotherapy with the vitamin C.

WS: How much vitamin C do you have her on?

HLN: Forty-eight grams a day in divided doses.

WS: And how large a woman is she?

HLN: She weighs around 118.

WS: That's not too terribly bad. I do think that if it were possible I would use some long-acting vitamin C at bedtime. You might add 7 grams that way.

HLN: Seven grams of the long-acting . . .

WS: She tolerates the regular ascorbic acid powder well?

HLN: Yes, she's on the straight ascorbic acid powder. I've used a lot of ascorbic acid for a long time for various other things. I tend to like the straight powder best.

WS: Better than the mixture of powdered ascorbic acid and sodium ascorbate?

HLN: Yes. Sooner or later it seems I have trouble with the sodium ascorbate with many patients. I usually use a straight ascorbic acid powder. It's a very fine powder that appears dull. I find that people don't tolerate the shiny powder well.

WS: I get the mixture of ascorbic acid and sodium ascorbate crystals.

HLN: Is it shiny or dull?

WS: It's fairly dull. It's not pure sodium ascorbate, which I think is a little high in sodium content for a lot of people.

---

* April 21, 1978.

HLN: Is it a 50–50 mixture?

WS: Yes, it comes out to a pH of about 6.* I found that a large number of people have been able to tolerate that.

HLN: Do you give it after meals or on an empty stomach?

WS: I have them take it after meals. As a matter of fact, I also have them take it in juice—raw vegetable juice or raw fruit juice—with no preservatives or sugar, of course.

HLN: You find that they tolerate the long-acting type fairly well, do you?

WS: Oh, yes, at bedtime.

HLN: You give them 7 grams at bedtime, is that right?

WS: Yes, I would advise 7 for your patient because of her size.

HLN: And how many hours does it last?

WS: Six hours. I have them start it first thing in the morning and keep it going all day long . . .

HLN: Have them start the other ascorbic acid, you mean?

WS: Yes.

HLN: And then have them take the long-acting just as they go to bed?

WS: As a bedtime adjunct. Now there's a physician who does not want his name used—you've probably heard of him—he also adds, in addition to megadoses of vitamin C, 200,000 units of vitamin A until they get a hair fall, and then backs off to 150,000 units, which stops the hair fall, he says. And he says that the vitamin A in combination with the vitamin C really shrinks tumors.

HLN: And he doesn't get any toxicity from that much vitamin A?

WS: Well, the initial manifestation of toxicity is the hair fall.

HLN: Sometimes you get cerebral symptoms from massive amounts of vitamin A, though.

---

* This is only slightly acid.

WS: Yes, but he hasn't been bothered with those.

HLN: Does he use the natural A?

WS: Yes.

HLN: Well, that's interesting. How many cancer patients have you treated?

WS: At the talk that I gave just a couple of months ago I reported that I treated 68. I know that 31 of them are alive. Twelve of them have just disappeared, moved away or something. I have no idea what's happened to them. The others have died. One of them, incidentally, was an oat cell carcinoma from Texas. I remember him very well.

HLN: The one that died?

WS: Yes.

HLN: Oat cell is supposed to respond fairly well to chemotherapy, as I understand it.

WS: Yes, well, he had the complete works of chemotherapy before he came to see me. And that's part of the bitter taste I got with chemotherapy.

HLN: Are you familiar with the Japanese who give chemotherapy and then give ascorbic acid a few minutes later? When I was in Scotland interviewing Cameron, he told me about it.

WS: That's interesting.

HLN: Do you recall what types of cancer you get most success with?

WS: Well, I've had real good success with renal carcinoma and fair success with various types other than oat cell. I've only got one girl with oat cell carcinoma that lived. Now she's been living since 1972, and she's doing very well. I have three of them that have various types of lymphoma and lymphosarcoma, one of them stage 4.

HLN: You've heard about Cameron's lymphosarcoma patient, I guess. He was given sodium ascorbate and the tumor disappeared in about a week. He stopped the vitamin C after about four or five months and the tumor came back. They gave him C again and the tumor went away again.

WS: I'll be darned.

HLN: Do you ever use calcium ascorbate?

68

WS: No. Jay Patrick has it out now, hideously expensive, and he has quite a bit of calcium in his. Calcium and potassium.

HLN: This patient of mine—do you think I ought to encourage her to go back into chemotherapy and continue her ascorbic acid?

WS: I don't know . . . Sounds interesting what you mentioned about the Japanese giving the ascorbic acid after chemotherapy—do they give it intravenously?

HLN: I'm not sure.

WS: I imagine that would be the best route to get to the cellular level.

HLN: What if this patient goes back into chemotherapy and gets too nauseated to take her ascorbic acid?

WS: Well, then she'll have to have it intravenously.

HLN: Just give it to her every day intravenously?

WS: Right. Would she be in a hospital setting?

HLN: No, she'd be an outpatient.

WS: Well, of course, if she can't continue it by mouth, then she'd have to stop the chemotherapy.

HLN: You would stop the chemotherapy if she couldn't take the ascorbic acid?

WS: Well, sure, because I think most of these people die of starvation, don't you?

HLN: Yes, I agree, that and intercurrent infections.

WS: Another interesting finding. I have found universally, regardless of what type of carcinoma they have, that these patients are either hypo- or achlorhydric,* and in order for them to get any nutrition you've got to supplement their acid.

HLN: I sometimes give ascorbic acid about an hour before meals. Some of my patients seem to tolerate it best that way. Maybe this supplies enough acid for the stomach.

WS: This patient that you have is taking 48 of pure ascorbic acid with a pH around 4, and has no G.I. [gastrointestinal] symptoms and is tolerating it well?

---

* Have little or no acid in their stomachs.

69

HLN: Yes. I have a patient in Dallas who takes 48 grams a day when he's feeling good, and if he feels bad he doubles it.

WS: That's amazing. You must have a real good source there.

HLN: I learned a lot when Linus Pauling's book came out a few years ago. Here in New York the stores sold out all their fine ascorbic acid powder and some of my patients switched over to the coarse, shiny ascorbic acid. I found that they did not do well on it. It was making them sick. Do you use the intravenous kind without a preservative?

WS: Right.

HLN: The sodium ascorbate?

WS: Yes, sodium ascorbate buffered to blood.

HLN: Well, is there any other advice you think I should give the general public?

WS: I would say that the most important thing that you could convey to them is to get back to the basics. There are a lot of screwy things in these health-food faddists and so forth, but to get to natural foods, well-cleaned vegetables, and to rule out the sugar—this is another thing that I think really is important.

HLN: Yes, I take all my patients off all processed foods.

WS: No preservatives, no artificial coloring and flavoring. In other words, eliminate the junk foods and get on natural foods. If the body isn't too terribly torn up it has the capacity of separating the wheat from the chaff.

HLN: I was on a radio talk show yesterday with a professor of nutrition. This is the second time we've been on together. I don't know why he goes on with me, because I give him such a hard time. Most people are afraid to go on with him, because he's got a lot of information, but I feel it's a lot of misinformation. He advocates that people eat sugar.

WS: Yes, isn't that the truth. And there's so much of it that's printed, too.

HLN: He really knows very little about clinical nutrition, doesn't even do research any more. He's just an administrator. But he's never worked much with patients, and he doesn't know much about human nutrition. It's really pitiful.

WS: Yes, this *is* pitiful, when they have such a wide swath of influence and no experience with real living, breathing people.

HLN: Well, I'm very grateful for your help. I appreciate your letting me use your experience in my book, and I appreciate your advice on this patient.

WS: Well, I wish you Godspeed, and I'm really thrilled and pleased to hear that somebody else has joined the ranks of us mavericks.

HLN: I don't think that there's anybody but you and myself who's using it in the States, so far as I know.

WS: Well, I'm certainly glad to hear that there's somebody there that I can refer people to.

8

Two Australian Doctors' Experience with Vitamin C for Cancer

No matter where you turn in the field of vitamin C, Irwin Stone's name keeps popping up. I learned that Stone has devised a new way of packaging injectable vitamin C. At present the sodium ascorbate designed for intravenous use comes already mixed with water, usually in 30-milliliter rubber-topped vials. Stone has devised a way to place sterile sodium ascorbate crystals in a vial. When ready to use the product, the physician simply mixes it with sterile water. This method saves shipping the large bottles containing the premixed ascorbate and insures that the solution will be full strength when used.

Stone employed the help of Dr. Glenn Dettman in Australia for the development of the product. When I spoke with Dr. Dettman about his work, he was most enthusiastic about both the product and the usefulness of vitamin C in the fight against cancer. Dettman is not a physician, so he gave me the name of two doctors in Australia who have had wide experience in the use of vitamin C to treat cancer.

The first is Dr. Archie Kalokerinos, of Mosman, New South Wales, who has treated something like 40 patients, almost all of whom were judged terminally ill and untreatable when they reached him.

The second Australian doctor is a delightful woman

who has treated over 50 patients and is quick to praise vitamin C. During our interview she told me that the medical society in her district was very uptight about physicians having their names in articles or books aimed at the general public. For this reason, she requested that I not use her real name, so I will call her "Dr. Lent."

INTERVIEW WITH DR. ARCHIE KALOKERINOS

H. L. NEWBOLD: Is vitamin C useful for treating cancer?

A. KALOKERINOS: It has a dramatic effect in relieving pain and making patients feel remarkably comfortable.

HLN: How many patients have you treated?

AK: Somewhere between 30 and 40.

HLN: Were these terminally ill patients?

AK: Yes, all of them.

HLN: Did they have other modalities of treatment prior to seeing you?

AK: Most of them did: surgery and radiation and chemotherapy.

HLN: How soon did the vitamin C bring pain relief?

AK: Usually it was a matter of a few days, sometimes two weeks.

HLN: How would you treat these patients?

AK: I used oral sodium ascorbate, gradually built them up to taking 8 grams four times a day. At the same time I gave supplements of B-group vitamins and zinc sulfate, about 200 milligrams per day.

HLN: Did you also give intravenous sodium ascorbate?

AK: Yes, for about a year I've been using intravenous of sodium ascorbate, between 30 and 60 grams intravenously three times a week.

HLN: You keep it up to control pain?

AK: The moment I stop the vitamin C injections

the tumors increase in size, so I use it to control the pain and to control the tumor size.

HLN: So you find that the amount of vitamin C they get determines the size of the tumor?

AK: Yes.

HLN: How effective has vitamin C been for reducing the size of the tumors?

AK: Well, the initial response with many of the patients is good. There was no apparent response in a few patients. Those patients rapidly deteriorated and died, but with many the initial response was quite good and the tumor definitely got smaller. All those who have been on treatment any length of time, however, had their tumors start to grow again.

HLN: After what length of time?

AK: Some of them after about six months.

HLN: Have you used large doses of vitamin A along with your program?

AK: Yes, I have on some, but not all. I am unable to determine whether vitamin A was of any benefit or not.

HLN: Any complications with vitamin C?

AK: A couple of patients hemorrhaged. When the tumors shrink they may pull on a blood vessel and cause a hemorrhage.

HLN: How serious have the hemorrhages been?

AK: It was fatal in one patient.

HLN: And you think it was due to the shrinkage of the cancer around the blood vessels?

AK: That is a possibility. The tumors were definitely getting smaller. The patient was feeling quite well.

HLN: Has anyone's life been saved by the use of vitamin C?

AK: Not in my hands. We are now treating a few patients that are not terminal. There was surgical removal of the first tumor, which was proven malignant, but no obvious signs of secondary invasion. I'm waiting to see if the effects of vitamin C here will be any better. Of course, we're going to have to wait an awful long time before we know the answer.

HLN: What diet do you encourage?

AK: Basically, I recommend good fresh food free of artificial preservatives, sweeteners, flavorings. I ask my patients to avoid white flour and sugar. I advocate mental relaxation for those who can be persuaded to practice it. Adequate rest is important, but patients should have some degree of physical activity if possible.

HLN: Do you find with vitamin C therapy people get up and start going about their activities again?

AK: Oh, yes, a great number.

HLN: So what you find is that vitamin C therapy prolongs their life and improves the quality of their life?

AK: Yes, very much so.

HLN: And have any of the patients you've treated been getting chemotherapy at the same time?

AK: Not the recent ones. A few years back some of them continued on the chemotherapy as well as the treatment I was giving.

HLN: Did you draw any conclusions about the compatibility of vitamin C therapy and chemotherapy?

AK: They are very compatible. If they are on my treatment and the chemotherapy, the chemotherapy doesn't have such harsh effects on them. They tolerate the chemotherapy better. Some doctors say giving the chemotherapy with the vitamin C may neutralize some of the effects of the chemotherapy.

HLN: What do you think of that?

AK: I'm not absolutely sure, but I feel that vitamin C would be helpful rather than harmful.

HLN: This is a question that always comes up— whether it protects the cancer cells as well as the healthy cells—but the consensus seems to be it's best to go ahead and take the ascorbic acid and the chemotherapy together.

AK: I couldn't argue with that. My experience is not great enough. I am fairly certain that we have to be careful with iron supplements. I believe that iron supplements can cause cancer in the first place, and if they are given to cancer patients they can do a great deal of harm.

HLN: What leads you to that conclusion?

AK: My conclusion comes from clinical observations, but now we have some theoretical reasons. You may have read it in *New Science* [December 1, 1977]. There's an article about zinc and iron, free radicals, in a recent edition of *Lancet,* giving some theoretical reasoning why iron supplements could be quite dangerous and why sorbate [vitamin C], vitamin E, and zinc would be helpful.

HLN: Zinc and selenium, maybe.

AK: Well, I don't think selenium is mentioned in any of these articles. I haven't gone too much into selenium. That is something we should go into a bit more closely. Some people have been suggesting that we shouldn't be giving nutritional supplements to cancer patients because it will help feed the cancer cells.

HLN: What do you think about that?

AK: Well, I never believed it.

HLN: I don't either.

AK: The patients feel so well while they're on vitamin C and other supplements that I haven't been able to deny them the benefit of it.

HLN: Yes, I agree that it's best to go ahead and give the supplements.

AK: That is what I do.

HLN: If patients are anemic, do you give them iron?

AK: If iron is going to be given, it should be in very small amounts. It should always be given in conjunction with vitamin C and zinc. Then the risks of iron supplements become much less.

HLN: So you would use it if you had a definite indication for it?

AK: Oh, yes, sometimes you've got to use iron, but I feel that the patients have to be really anemic before I use it.

HLN: Do you treat any leukemias?

AK: Yes.

HLN: What kind of results have you had?

AK: So far I've only treated one and it was terminal. He had a very rapid termination.

HLN: What impression do you have about certain

types of tumors doing better than others with vitamin C?

AK: Certain patients have done better than others. I haven't been able to give any explanation for this.

HLN: Have you treated any oat cell carcinoma of the lung?

AK: Yes.

HLN: What happened?

AK: It was rapidly fatal.

HLN: I have one I'm treating now. She was on chemotherapy and got disgusted with it and stopped. They thought she was going to die in December, but she's still doing beautifully. I keep my fingers crossed. How much vitamin A do you give when you use it?

AK: Something like 1,000 units a day.

HLN: This patient of mine with the oat cell carcinoma of the lung was on 200,000 units a day of vitamin A when she began to become a little toxic, depressed and weepy. We had to go down to 150,000. She was on zinc, too, 180 milligrams a day of zinc gluconate. Do you give folic acid anytime?

AK: I've never given it to cancer patients. I use it a lot in elderly people. We've done a lot of folic acid blood studies, which often show low levels. But I haven't used folic acid routinely.

HLN: What about vitamin B_{12}?

AK: I don't rely too much on blood levels and all the strict clinical signs. If I think it's needed, I give it; otherwise you might lose a year or two waiting for clinical signs of deficiency to present themselves.

HLN: Anything else the general public should know about vitamin C and cancer?

AK: Well, there's the preventive role. I would rather try to prevent cancer by using large doses of vitamin C.

HLN: How much do you think people should take as a preventive?

AK: It would naturally vary from person to person, but an average for an adult should be 10 grams a day.

HLN: Do you have any statistics on that?

AK: No, but I've got a lot of people taking it.

HLN: Have you treated any skin cancer with vitamin C ointment?

AK: Yes.

HLN: What kind of results did you have?

AK: Very, very good.

HLN: What percentage ointment do you use?

AK: I make a 50–50 mixture, 50 percent sodium sorbate powder in an ointment base.

HLN: That's 50–50 by weight?

AK: I mix it up pretty roughly myself.

HLN: Did you do it by weight or by volume?

AK: I would say by volume.

HLN: And you use the sodium ascorbate?

AK: Yes.

HLN: Then how often do patients apply it?

AK: Very frequently. I try to get them to put it on six times a day.

HLN: How many skin cancers have you treated?

AK: I would say about half a dozen.

HLN: Some of them were advanced?

AK: No, none of them were what you would call really advanced.

HLN: And what kind of results did you get?

AK: They just shriveled up.

HLN: How long did it take?

AK: Six months.

HLN: Did you give them vitamin C by mouth also?

AK: Yes.

HLN: I've had very good results with using vitamin C ointment locally also. I get results in less than six months, though. I've used the straight ascorbic acid, 30 percent by weight. Do you keep the ointment in the refrigerator?

AK: No, I mix it up each time fresh. I don't tell them to put it in the refrigerator. Maybe I should.

HLN: How often do they get a new supply of it?

AK: It generally only lasts about a week.

HLN: So it's pretty fresh all the time.

AK: The sodium ascorbate ointment becomes hydroscopic and absorbs a lot of water and stuff . . .

HLN: Anything else?

78

AK: Just don't write that I say vitamin C will cure all types of cancer. It will cure skin cancer. Other types of cancer are often made to shrink. Patients feel better and live longer, but I haven't seen anyone with cancer get free of the cancer once it has spread.

INTERVIEW WITH DR. LENT

H. L. NEWBOLD: This is Dr. Newbold in New York. Your name was given to me by Dr. Dettman. I am writing a book on the use of vitamin C for cancer, and I understand that you've done some work in that area.

LENT: Yes, I've done a lot of work in that area.

HLN: How many cancer patients have you treated with ascorbic acid?

L: Maybe 50.

HLN: That's quite an experience.

L: It could be a bit more.

HLN: What are your impressions about it?

L: Vitamin C is absolutely super as a painkiller. It's absolutely smashing. Often within a few seconds after giving a high dose of vitamin C the pain is under control.

HLN: How much vitamin C?

L: I give 30 grams in half a liter.

HLN: Do you use Ringer's lactate or sodium chloride?

L: Sodium chloride is perfectly satisfactory.

HLN: Over what period of time do you let it run in?

L: Well, I just let it run itself out. It generally takes a half to three quarters of an hour. Right now I have a man with cancer that I've been giving 60 grams.

HLN: Why do you give him 60 instead of 30 grams?

L: Well, I found that 60 grams is what he needs to control his pain.

HLN: You cannot put 60 grams in five hundred cc's?

L: Sixty grams in 1 liter.

79

HLN: Would it work to put 60 grams in half a liter?

L: No, because it's too strong that way and hurts the veins.

HLN: How often do you give that intravenously?

L: Well, I start off giving 30 grams a day for ten days; then I begin spreading it out according to how much pain the patient has.

HLN: Do you find that you get much better relief by giving it intravenously rather than by the mouth?

L: I can't quite give the same high dosages to the mouth. They get diarrhea.

HLN: Do patients regularly take vitamin C by mouth even though they are getting it intravenously?

L: Yes, I build it up as high as they can tolerate by mouth.

HLN: Do you use the sodium ascorbate or ascorbic acid?

L: Sodium ascorbate.

HLN: Do you have any trouble with the sodium ion?

L: The only trouble is that the patients get extremely thirsty. We let them drink all they want.

HLN: Do they retain fluids?

L: No.

HLN: Are the patients you see terminally ill?

L: Oh, yes, they all had terminal cancers. They had all been given up for dead.

HLN: Have they all had chemotherapy and X ray and everything?

L: Some of them have and some of them haven't.

HLN: Do you feel that you're prolonging their lives?

L: Yes.

HLN: Do you have any impressions on what types of tumors you get best results with?

L: We don't seem to have good luck with lung cancers.

HLN: Do you use large dosages of vitamin A also?

L: No, I don't. I haven't gone into that yet.

HLN: Do you use zinc?

L: No.

HLN: Do you advise special diets?

L: Yes, I do.

HLN: What?

L: I put them on fruits and vegetables and whole-bran cereals.

HLN: Why do you do that?

L: That's the diet most doctors use who are treating cancer patients this way.

HLN: Is there anything else the general public should know about this subject?

L: About vitamin C in the treatment of cancer?

HLN: Yes.

L: Just that I think that vitamin C is very, very helpful in treating cancer.

9

The Vitamin C Guru: Irwin Stone

There is no question that Irwin Stone knows more about vitamin C than anyone else in the world. All of us who have been especially interested in that vitamin have looked upon him as the guru.

We didn't get off to a very good start. About five years ago I was on a speaking program with him in New York. Before the meeting we had dinner together with a number of other people. He wanted me to try some of his vitamin C powder, which he had mixed with table sugar. When I balked, he more or less insisted. I had my own vitamin C powder and chose to use it. Since I am allergic to sugar, I naturally avoid it. I feel that for many reasons everyone should avoid sugar.

Be that as it may, I am well aware that Irwin Stone knows more about vitamin C than anyone else in the world and I am very grateful to him for the time and advice he has given me while compiling this book.

INTERVIEW WITH IRWIN STONE

H. L. NEWBOLD: I understand you were the one who got Linus Pauling interested in vitamin C.

I. STONE: I attended a meeting in New York in March of 1966 of the Carl Neuberg Society, where Linus Pauling was giving a talk. During the course of the talk he mentioned that he'd like to live about fifteen more years to see the results of his research. I tried to see him at the meeting, but he was surrounded by so many people I couldn't get close to him. So I wrote a letter that told him that I had been working with ascorbic acid since 1934 and that I had developed some unique theories about it, and I sent him a copy of my megascorbic regimen.

I told him if he went on ascorbic acid he would not only live fifteen more years but he would probably live an additional fifty years.

I also included the regimen that I had worked out for preventing and treating the common cold. The information hit him at the right time, because he was formulating his ideas on orthomolecular medicine. Both Dr. Pauling and his wife tried out my cold regimen and found it worked.

Also, I think it was just about that time that he broke his leg and found that when he took the vitamin C his leg healed much more rapidly than anyone had expected.

I think it was at a dedication at Mount Sinai Hospital in New York that he mentioned that the ascorbic acid was very useful in preventing and treating the common cold. That started a big row with the medical profession. The doctors jumped on him and told him he was crazy.

He then looked up the literature on the use of vitamin C in the treatment of the common cold and found that a lot of tests had been done, which everybody had ignored. He then took off three or four months and wrote his first book, *Vitamin C and the Common Cold,* and dedicated the book to me and Szent-Györgyi, and that's how it all started.

HLN: Rumor has it that Pauling was about ready to retire and sit out in the backwaters of life until he started taking vitamin C.

IS: No, I don't think that was the case, because when he retired from Stanford he had his institute already going. It was located right outside the Stanford campus, in Menlo Park.

HLN: What is the earliest use of vitamin C to treat cancer?

IS: It's in my book.* It probably goes back to around 1936, way back.

HLN: I have just been over to Scotland talking to Cameron, who is doing some interesting work, which I'm sure you're familiar with. He's using 10 grams of ascorbic acid.

IS: I think Cameron is using too little ascorbate for effective results.

HLN: Yes, I agree with you. How much do you think should be used?

IS: Oh, anywhere from 50 to 100 grams.

HLN: Has anybody taken that dose over a long period of time?

IS: Well, it's been used in cancer and Dr. [name deleted] has used up to 300 grams a day in the treatment of viral diseases.

HLN: Yes, but that was for short periods of time.

IS: Yes, it usually cures the disease in three days.

HLN: How long do you think the cancer treatment should go on?

IS: Well, it depends on the response of the patient. I think ascorbate should always be in association with the other therapy. The ascorbate will keep the patient alive.

HLN: A question comes up about using vitamin C with chemotherapy in the treatment of cancer. Will vitamin C detoxify the chemotherapeutic agent and protect the cancer cells as well as the healthy cells?

IS: There was a paper from the National Cancer Institute in 1969 which showed that ascorbate killed cancer cells and didn't affect the normal cells, so it has its own chemotherapeutic action even though it isn't toxic.

HLN: Yes, I understand that. What do you think about using it in conjunction with chemotherapy?

_____

* *The Healing Factor: Vitamin C Against Disease.* New York: Grosset & Dunlap, 1972.

IS: It should always be used, because it permits the survival of the patient.

HLN: What about this theoretical objection that it may protect the cancer from the chemotherapy?

IS: I don't think that's a valid objection, though I don't have much experimental evidence to back me up. But I think it should always be used, with radiation therapy also. It protects the patient.

HLN: Certainly the patients are more comfortable with it.

IS: You see, all these patients have a severe case of chronic subclinical scurvy.

HLN: I think it's almost a universal disease.

IS: It is, because there's no protection against this genetic defect.

HLN: I have a patient from Dallas who flies up to see me. He takes 48 grams a day regularly, and when he feels bad he doubles it.

IS: Yes, well, that's been the case. Have you seen my paper on leukemia?

HLN: No, I don't believe so.

IS: It's not the leukemia that kills the patient. It's either hemorrhage or infection, and hemorrhage and infection are pathognomonic symptoms of scurvy. So if you correct the scurvy at least the patient has half a chance to survive.

HLN: When you say 50 to 100 grams a day, do you mean over the remainder of the patient's lifetime?

IS: Well, I don't think it would be necessary, but you have to see how the patient responds. We've been using sodium ascorbate for drug addiction. During the active stages of treatment we usually give about 20 to 80 grams a day, usually 30 to 40 grams.

HLN: That's just for a few days, though.

IS: We give it for about a week, and then we reduce it to holding doses of about 10 grams sodium ascorbate a day. The patients stay on that for the rest of their lives with the multivitamins and minerals.

HLN: Do you think cancer patients should be treated the same way?

IS: Cancer patients should be treated the same way.

You have to give them the high doses until they show some kind of improvement.

HLN: Would you do it intravenously or all by mouth?

IS: Give it both ways. During the work we [Dr. William Saccoman and Stone] did in San Diego on cancer we started the patient off on 50 grams a day. We gave 30 grams of that intravenously and about 20 orally. Then we gradually reduced the intravenous but maintained a total of 50 grams a day by mouth. At the end of two weeks we had them off the intravenous. They were all on oral, and we continued that until they showed signs of recovery.

HLN: These were cancer patients?

IS: Yes. Now in one case we treated Hodgkin's disease. We gave the patient 30 grams a day for the last three years. The patient shows no signs of the disease any more, but we still keep her on the 30 grams a day just to be sure and to keep her free of chronic subclinical scurvy.

HLN: Is this the sodium ascorbate or the straight ascorbic acid?

IS: It's a mixture.

HLN: Why a mixture?

IS: Well, because some of them don't want to take it with sodium, and I don't like to give too much of the ascorbic acid because it may cause gastric distress.

HLN: Do you give it on empty stomach or after meals?

IS: They've been taking it with their meals.

HLN: Have you ever tried it on an empty stomach?

IS: Yes, that was the way we were doing it at first with the ascorbic acid, but we found that we got a lot of gastric distress that way because of the high acidity, so we reduced it by using the sodium ascorbate, because it is not acid. It's tasteless, so you can put it in any food.*

HLN: Why sodium instead of calcium ascorbate?

---

* He used a different brand of ascorbic acid from the one I prescribe, hence our experience differs.

86

IS: At the time calcium wasn't available. It's available now, but I don't like to give too much calcium. Right now we use a mixture of sodium and calcium.

HLN: You think it doesn't make any difference in terms of the physiological effect?

IS: Usually these patients can handle it. When they're on these high levels of ascorbate they have a better tolerance of sodium.

HLN: How did you originally get interested in vitamin C?

IS: I've been working with ascorbate since 1934. I first worked in the chemical technology of ascorbic acid. I started two years after it was discovered. I was working in a chemical research laboratory. It all started with beer. We were investigating the stability of beer, trying to improve it. I thought we could use ascorbic acid to improve the stability and improve the flavor of beer, and it worked. So we got the first U.S. patent to use ascorbic acid to stabilize beer. That's how it all started. In 1939 or 1940 I got interested in the clinical aspects of vitamin C.

HLN: What are you busy with now?

IS: I'm still working with megascorbics. I've spent my whole life on it.

HLN: What aspect now?

IS: Trying to clear up the almost universal chronic subclinical scurvy, which is epidemic in the population.

HLN: How do you go about this?

IS: I lecture, I do research and write scientific papers for publication, and I'm a member of the Linus Pauling Institute, so I keep very busy. It is an educational job and I try to interest younger members of the profession to undertake clinical research in the many unexplored areas of megascorbic therapy.

The following is a chapter from Irwin Stone's book *The Healing Factor: Vitamin C Against Disease.*

Cancer
By Irwin Stone

Over half a million people in the United States develop cancer each year and over 280,000 will die of cancer in the year ahead. More than 700,000 people are under treatment at all times. It is the number two scourge and one of every five of us is likely to be afflicted; under present conditions it will send one of every eight of us to the grave.

Cancer is not a single disease but a large group of closely related, yet different, diseases. Essentially, cancerous growth is uncontrolled tissue development and expansion and is due to the tissue losing the normal restraints on cell division and growth. The cancer grows in a wild manner at the expense of the surrounding normal tissues. Cancer can arise in any organ or tissue of the body and, like the infectious diseases, the causes are varied and different. In severity it can range from a relatively innocuous minor illness to a life-threatening disease. The pattern of cancer incidence has been changing over the years, with fewer stomach and uterine cancers and more lung cancer and leukemia.

Present-Day Cancer Therapy

In the therapy of cancer, the first important step is diagnosis. After diagnosis, the physician has three different paths or a combination of them from which to choose: irradiation, chemotherapy, or surgery. Irradiation is localized exposure to X rays or to the radiant energy of radioactive sources, such as radium or cobalt 60, to try to kill the fast-growing cancerous tissue without doing too much damage to the rest of the body. Chemotherapy involves the use of chemical substances that tend to damage the cancer tissue more than the normal cells and thus retard the cancer development. Surgery, of course, is the direct approach of going in and physically removing the cancerous tissue, when possible.

Ever since the discovery of ascorbic acid in the early

1930's, there has been a vast amount of animal experimentation and clinical research conducted on the relationship of ascorbic acid to cancer. This has resulted in a mass of conflicting and confusing reports as to the value of ascorbic acid in cancer treatments. Some investigators reported good results in their tests, others reported no effects on the growth of cancer tissue, while still others took the stand that it stimulated tumor growth. Detailed discussion of the possible reasons for the conflicts of opinion in this work is beyond the scope of this chapter, except to speculate that it may be due to the wide variety of experimental animals, cancer types, and experimental conditions employed by the numerous investigators. As a first step in future cancer research on ascorbic acid, a responsible, unbiased research agency should review this large volume of early work and assess its value in the light of the more recent research and newer concepts. Any research work which may be required to resolve these unanswered questions and conflicting opinions should be conducted. Because of the long-standing disagreement and the resulting confusion, there has probably been a tendency for research workers to shy away from this area.

One thing, however, is certain. Cancer and its present-day therapy are intense biochemical stresses which deplete the bodies of cancer victims of their ascorbic acid. The irradiation, the surgery, or the chemotherapy with highly toxic materials are all severe biochemical stresses. Biochemical stresses, in the majority of the mammals which are able to produce their own ascorbic acid, cause them to produce more ascorbic acid to combat the stresses. Because of their defective genetic inheritance, mammals such as guinea pigs, monkeys, and man are dependent on their food intake for ascorbic acid and their response to stress is ascorbic acid depletion.

Experiments on rats, mice, and guinea pigs are enlightening on this point. When rats and mice (animals that can make their own ascorbic acid) are exposed to cancer-producing agents (carcinogens), they start producing much more ascorbic acid in their livers.[1] However, when guinea pigs (animals which, like man, cannot produce their own ascorbic acid) are exposed to the same carcinogens, their ascorbic acid is used up and not replaced;[2]

to quote the authors of this 1955 paper, when mammals are exposed to carcinogens this will "excite an increased demand for this compound (ascorbic acid) to which the animals capable of synthesizing it respond by overproduction, whereas in those lacking this power the store is depleted."

In another experiment on guinea pigs, Russell,[3] in 1952, showed that cancers developed sooner in guinea pigs exposed to carcinogens and fed a diet deficient in ascorbic acid as compared to guinea pigs exposed to the same carcinogens but on an adequate ascorbic acid diet. Can we extrapolate this observation to humans and say that people who do not fully "correct" their genetic disease, hypoascorbemia, by continuously taking high levels of ascorbic acid are more susceptible to cancer than fully "corrected" individuals?

An opposite view is taken in the 1955 paper by Miller and Sokoloff,[3] who proposed that a prescorbutic state in the cancer victim may have beneficial effects on cancer patients during radiation therapy. To settle this question once and for all should not entail much additional research. A person afflicted with cancer will almost always be nearly depleted of ascorbic acid before the usual course of therapy is begun. Radiation therapy using radiant energy in the form of X rays or gamma rays is a potent form of biochemical stress for the body. Exposing a cancer victim to radiant energy only further aggravates a serious shortage of this metabolite and prevents the body from maintaining biochemical homeostasis under the onslaughts of the additional radiation stresses. There have been other papers published which suggested giving ascorbic acid to cancer patients before exposure to radiation and noting its benefits.[4] In spite of these many suggestions, further large-scale conclusive research has not been conducted and the practice is little used. These scientists, in their clinical work, used, at most, a few grams of ascorbic acid a day. The full correction of the combined stresses of the cancer and the radiation may need much higher doses of ascorbic acid each day. This is another virgin area of megascorbic therapy, just awaiting someone to go in and try it.

Cancer chemotherapy is the use of certain chemicals to

selectively poison the cancer cells without killing the patient. We will not go into the chemistry of the different materials used other than to say that they are all very poisonous and dangerous (host toxic). This, of course, limits the amounts which can be given the patient at any one time. One group of materials used in cancer chemotherapy is the so-called nitrogen mustards, which are derivatives of the mustard gases of World War I; you can conceive the type of material used in this therapy. While the chemotherapeutic agent will attack the cancer cells, the patient is left without means to overcome the toxic manifestations of the medicament. In spite of the fact that ascorbic acid has been known to be an efficient detoxicating agent for poisonous substances no reports have been found in the medical literature for the combined administration of these toxic medicaments along with large doses of ascorbic acid as a supportive measure. The presence of high optimal levels of ascorbic acid might also improve the toxic action on the cancer cells [5], but we will never know it unless it is thoroughly investigated. The potential benefits, if successful, would seem to make these clinical trials an urgent necessity.

The data contained in the 1969 paper from Dean Burk and his group [5] at the National Cancer Institute are very pertinent at this point. They showed that ascorbate is highly toxic to the cancer cells they used (Ehrlich ascites carcinoma cells) and caused profound structural changes in the cancer cells in their laboratory cultures. They mention that:

> The great advantage that ascorbates . . . possess as potential anticancer agents is that they are, like penicillin, remarkably nontoxic to normal body tissues, and they may be administered to animals in extremely large doses (up to 5 or more grams per kilogram) without notable harmful pharmacological effects.

5 grams per kilogram on a 70-kilogram adult would amount to 350 grams of ascorbic acid per day. They further state:

> In our view, the future of effective cancer chemo-

therapy will not rest on the use of host-toxic compounds now so widely employed, but upon virtually host-non-toxic compounds that are lethal to cancer cells, of which ascorbate . . . represents an excellent prototype example.

They also bring out the amazing fact that in the screening program that has been going on for years to find new cancer-killing materials at the Cancer Chemotherapy National Service Center, ascorbic acid has been bypassed, excluded from consideration, and never tested for its cancer-killing properties. The reason given for not screening ascorbic acid is even more fantastic—ascorbic acid was too nontoxic to fit into their program!

An almost immediate confirmation of Dean Burk's proposals was contained in the research conducted at Tulane University School of Medicine by Schlegel and coworkers and published in 1969.[5] It was shown that bladder cancer due to smoking and other causes could be prevented by ascorbic acid. They recommended the intake of 1.5 grams of ascorbic acid a day to avoid the recurrence of bladder tumors.

The remaining area of cancer therapy, surgery, is one where ascorbic acid may now be used to some extent. It may be used, not so much for its direct effect on the cancer, but for its beneficial effects in wound healing. For this purpose it is generally used at a gram or so a day, which may be quite inadequate to handle the biochemical stresses of anesthesia, surgical shock, and hemorrhagic shock on an already depleted cancer victim. Full "correction" of the victim's hypoascorbemia may require instituting a preoperative, operative, and postoperative regime at much higher levels. Additional research on a regime of this sort may uncover possibilities for survival and cure far beyond today's hopes.

Use of Ascorbic Acid in Cancer Therapy

Present-day cancer therapy thus virtually ignores the potential of ascorbic acid as a biochemical stress combatant, a detoxicant, an anticarcinogenic agent, a means for maintaining homeostasis, and a mechanism for improving the well-being and survival of the patient.

During the past forty years there have been many papers published in the medical literature on which ascorbic acid has been used for cancer therapy. But no one in all this time has consistently used ascorbic acid in the large doses which may be required to demonstrate a therapeutic effect. There has never been a well-planned program to test ascorbic acid in cancer therapy and no one has used more than a gram or, at most, several grams a day (except in one case, discussed later).

Deucher,[4] in 1940, used up to 4 grams of ascorbic acid a day for several days in treating his cancer patients and found it had a remarkably favorable effect on their general condition and increased their tolerance to X rays. On the other hand, Szenes,[4] in 1942, stated that the administration of ascorbic acid is contraindicated in tumor patients because it intensifies tumor growth.

It was also used in combination with vitamin A, which only further complicated the picture, in a series of tests. Von Wendt, in 1949, 1950, and 1951, and Huber, in 1953, used 2 grams of ascorbic acid a day combined with large doses of vitamin A and reported favorable effects. Schneider, in 1954, 1955, and 1956, also used ascorbic acid, 1 gram daily in combination with vitamin A, and found that it "arrested" cancers, that it was more useful against epitheliomas than against sarcomas.[6]

Of interest also are three papers by McCormick,[7] in 1954, 1959, and 1963, in which he postulates the theory that the factor which preconditions the body to the development of cancer is the degenerative changes caused by continued low levels of ascorbic acid in the body. He gives evidence to support his hypothesis and states, "We maintain that the degree of malignancy is determined inversely by the degree of connective tissue resistance, which in turn is dependent upon the adequacy of vitamin C status." McCormick's ideas have never been adequately tested.

Some additional evidence for the support of this hypothesis comes from the work of Goth and Littmann,[8] in 1948, who found that cancers most frequently originate in organs whose ascorbic acid levels are below 4.5 mg% and rarely grow in organs containing ascorbic acid above this concentration. Fully corrected individuals should have tissue levels of ascorbic acid in excess of this seemingly critical 4.5 mg%.

Detoxication of Carcinogens

Another piece of research which has not been properly followed through was reported by Warren,[9] in 1943, who showed that certain carcinogens, anthracene, and 3:4-benzpyrene (the type of carcinogen in tobacco smoke), are susceptible to oxidation in the presence of ascorbic acid. In the oxidized form they are no longer carcinogenic.

Here is a possible means for preventing the induction of cancer after exposure to carcinogens merely by maintaining the necessary levels of ascorbic acid in the exposed tissues. This is an area of research that has been stagnant for two decades, which would have the most important consequences for smokers or city dwellers forced to breathe polluted air, or for others exposed to carcinogens.

Leukemia

Leukemia is a cancerous disease of the blood-forming tissues in which there is an overproduction of the white blood cells (leukocytes). Different types of leukemia are named after the different varieties of leukocytes involved in the disease process. The overproduction of the leukocytes causes, in most cases, a marked rise in the numbers of white blood cells in the circulating blood.

Research work connecting ascorbic acid, the blood elements, and leukemia was started not long after the discovery of ascorbic acid. Stephen and Hawley,[10] in 1936, showed that when the blood was separated into plasma, red blood cells, and white blood cells, there was a 20- to 30-fold concentration of ascorbic acid in the white blood cells.

Hemorrhage, being a symptom of both leukemia and scurvy, caused clinicians to early investigate the use of ascorbic acid in leukemia because of its dramatic effects on hemorrhage in scurvy. Eufinger and Gaehtgens,[11] in 1936, reported giving 200 milligrams of ascorbic acid a day and came to the conclusion that it had a normalizing influence on the blood picture. Schnetz,[11] in 1940, came to the same conclusion: when the leukocytes are high ascorbic acid tends to reduce them, and when they are low it tends to increase them. He used 200 to 900 milligrams a day by injection.

Here is a marked example of the ancient mammalian mechanism of ascorbic acid homeostasis.

In 1936, Plum and Thomsen,[12] injecting 200 milligrams of ascorbic acid a day, obtained remissions in two cases of myeloid leukemia, and Heinild and Schiedt,[12] using two 100-milligram injections daily, obtained uncertain, variable results. Thiele,[12] in 1938, using 500 milligrams of ascorbic acid a day by injection, found no effect in chronic myeloid leukemia, while both Palenque [4] and van Nieuwenhuizen,[12] in 1943, observed slight decreases in the white blood counts. Such variable and confusing results are typical when submarginal and inadequate dosages are employed.

Vogt, in 1940, in a review of the work conducted on ascorbic acid in leukemia up to that time, cited twenty-one references. About the only conclusion he reached was that there were high deficits of ascorbic acid in leukemics. These deficits and the very low blood plasma levels of ascorbic acid in leukemics were confirmed in later papers by Kyhos et al., in 1945, and Waldo and Zipf, in 1955, and yet, in all these years, no one was inspired to get away from these pitifully small doses of ascorbic acid and make some clinical tests with heroic doses.[13]

In a leukemic, the biochemical stresses of the disease process has reduced the body stores of ascorbic acid to very low levels. Any ascorbic acid circulating in the blood has been scavenged and locked in the excessive numbers of the white blood cells contained in the blood. The plasma level of ascorbic acid is usually zero or close thereto. A zero level in the blood plasma means that the tissues of the body are not being supplied with this most important metabolite. The ascorbic acid contained in the leukocytes are unavailable for the tissues. The tissues are in a condition of biochemical scurvy and this explains why these depleted tissues are so susceptible to the characteristic hemorrhaging of leukemia and the infections that kill so many of the leukemics. A leukemic is not only suffering from leukemia but also from a bad case of biochemical scurvy. To correct this condition, ascorbic acid has to be administered in sufficiently large doses not only to saturate the excess of white blood cells but to provide adequate spillover into the blood plasma and tissues so that the seriously ill leukemic will be given a fighting chance to combat the disease. This may require the administration of ascorbic acid at the rate of 25 or more grams per day, as noted in the following case of leukemia treated with megascorbic levels of ascorbic acid.

This case history, reported by Greer,[14] in 1954, was of a seventy-one-year-old executive of an oil company, who was first seen for alcoholic cirrhosis of the liver and polycythemia (excess of red blood cells); some months earlier, symptoms of chronic myocarditis had appeared. Shortly thereafter, he was hospitalized and passed a large uric acid bladder stone, and a diagnosis of chronic myelogenous leukemia was established. He also had intractable pyorrhea and his remaining 17 teeth were removed at one operation. At this time he started taking ascorbic acid at the rate of 24.5 grams to 42 grams per day, "because he reported he felt much better when he took these large doses." Since the diagnosis of leukemia and the removal of the teeth, "the patient has repeatedly remarked about his feeling of well-being and has continued his vocation as executive of an oil company." On two occasions, at the insistence of his attending physician, he stopped taking the ascorbic acid and both times his spleen and liver enlarged and became tender, his temperature rose to 101°, and he complained of general malaise and fatigue (typical leukemia symptoms). When he started the ascorbic acid again, the symptoms cleared and his temperature became normal within 6 hours. Over a year and a half later the patient had a severe attack of epidemic diarrhea and died of acute cardiac decompensation. At the time of death, the spleen was firm, not tender, and had not enlarged since taking of ascorbic acid. The doctor also reported that "the polycythemia, leukemia, cirrhosis, and the myocarditis had shown no progression" in the year and a half while taking the ascorbic acid. The case history concludes with the statement, "The intake of the huge doses of ascorbic acid appeared essential for the welfare of the patient."

One would believe that the exciting results in this 1954 case would be immediately picked up and explored further by the leukemia groups in the national government or the foundations that are continually asking the public for more research money, but no follow-up work has been found in the medical literature of the past sixteen years. If megascorbic therapy could do so much for an aged leukemic with so many other complications, what could it do for the young, uncomplicated leukemic? The answer to this question could be obtained easily and each day lost may mean more lives wasted. At the present time, millions of dollars are spent in screening all sorts of poisonous chemicals for use in leukemia, while a harmless substance like ascorbic acid, with so much potential, lies around neglected and ignored.

Recent work has brought forward evidence that human leukemia may be caused by a virus. While viruses are known to produce cancer-like diseases in animals, none have been proved in man. If the cause of human leukemia is eventually shown to be due to a virus, the rationale for the use of megascorbic therapy in leukemia will be further strengthened because it has been shown that ascorbic acid is a potent, wide-spectrum, nontoxic virucide when used at megascorbic dosage levels.

NOTES

1. E. L. Kennaway et al., "Effect of Aromatic Compounds upon the Ascorbic Acid Content of the Liver in Mice," *Cancer Research,* vol. 4, pp. 367–376, 1944.

M. Daff et al., "Effect of Carcinogenic Compounds on the Ascorbic Acid Content of the Liver in Mice and Rats," *Cancer Research,* vol. 8, pp. 376–380, 1948.

L. A. Elson et al., "Effect of 1:2:5:6 Dibenzanthrene on the Ascorbic Acid Content of the Liver of Rats Maintained on High and Low Protein Diets," *British Journal of Cancer,* vol. 3, pp. 148–156, 1949.

E. Boyland et al., "Stimulation of Ascorbic Acid Synthesis by Carcinogenic and Other Foreign Compounds," *Biochemical Journal,* vol. 81, pp, 163–168, 1961.

2. E. L. Kennaway et al., "Carcinogenic Agents and the Metabolism of Ascorbic Acid in the Guinea Pig," *British Journal of Cancer,* vol. 9, pp. 606–610, 1955.

3. W. O. Russell et al., "Studies on Methylcholanthrene Induction of Tumors in Scorbutic Guinea Pigs," *Cancer Research,* vol. 12, pp. 216–218, 1952.

T. R. Miller and B. Sokoloff, "A Vitamin C–Free Diet in Radiation Therapy of Malignant Disease," *Journal of Roentgenology,* vol. 73, pp. 472–480, 1955.

4. W. G. Deucher, "Vitamin C Metabolism in Tumor Patients," *Strahlentherapie,* vol. 67, pp. 143–151, 1940.

E. Palenque, "On the Treatment of Chronic Myeloid Leukemia with Vitamin C," *Semana Medica Espanola,* vol. 6, pp. 101–105, 1943.

H. Schirmacher and J. Schneider, "Limits and Possibilities of Supervitaminization for Inoperable and X-ray Resistant Carcinoma," *Zeitschrift fur Geburtshilfe und Gyanaekologie* (Stuttgart), vol. 144, pp. 172–182, 1955.

E. Piche and K. Weghaupt, "Treatment of Advanced Carcinomas of Female Genitalia with Large Doses of Vitamin A and C," *Wiener Medizinische Wochenschrift,* vol. 106, pp. 391–392, 1956.

S. B. Tagi-Zade, "Vitamin C Metabolism in Cancer Patients During Radiotherapy," *Meditsinskaia Radiologiia* (Moskva), vol. 6, pp. 10–16, 1961.

T. Szenes, "Effect Of Ascorbic Acid During Roentgen Irradiation Of Tumors," *Strahlentherapie,* vol. 71, pp. 463–471, 1942.

5. L. Benade, T. Howard and D. Burk, "Synergistic Killing of Ehrlich Ascites Carcinoma Cells by Ascorbate and 3-Amino-1,2,4-Triazole," *Oncology,* vol. 23, pp. 33–43, 1969.

J. U. Schlegel et al., "Studies in the Etiology and Prevention of Bladder Carcinoma," *The Journal of Urology,* vol. 101, pp. 317–324, 1969.

6. von Wendt, *Zeitschrift fur die Gesamte Innere Medizin und Ihre Grenzgebiete* (Stuttgart), vol. 4, p. 267, 1949; vol. 5, p. 255, 1950; vol. 6, pp. 255–256, 1951; *Hippokrates* (Stuttgart), H. 9, 1951.

L. Huber, "Hypervitaminization with Vitamin A and Vitamin C: In Cases of Inoperable Cancer of the Uterus,"

Zentralblatt fur Gynaekologie, vol. 75, pp. 1771–1777, 1953.

E. Schneider, "Vitamin C and A in Cancer," *Deutsche Medizinische Wochenshrift*, vol. 79, pp. 584–586, 1954; "Mechanism of Resistance to Cancer Shown by a Skin Reaction," *Wiener Medizinische Wochenschrift*, vol. 105, pp. 430–432, 1955; "Hypervitamin Therapy of Cancer," *Medizinische*, pp. 183–187, 1956.

7. W. J. McCormick, "Cancer: The Preconditioning Factor in Pathogenesis," *Archives of Pediatrics*, vol. 71, pp. 313–322, 1954; "Cancer: A Collagen Disease, Secondary to a Nutritional Deficiency?" *ibid.*, vol. 76, pp. 166–171, 1959; "Cancer: A Preventable Disease, Secondary to a Nutritional Deficiency," *Clinical Physiology*, vol. 5, pp. 198–204, 1963.

8. A. Goth and I. Littmann, "Ascorbic Acid Content in Human Cancer Tissue," *Cancer Research*, vol. 8, pp. 349–351, 1948.

9. F. L. Warren, "Aerobic Oxidation of Aromatic Hydrocarbons in Presence of Ascorbic Acid," *Biochemical Journal*, vol. 37, pp. 338–341, 1943.

10. D. J. Stephen and E. E. Hawley, "Portion of Reduced Ascorbic Acid in Blood," *Journal of Biological Chemistry*, vol. 115, pp. 653–658, 1936.

11. H. Eufinger and G. Gaehtgens, "Effect of Vitamin C on the Pathologic Concentrations of White Blood Cells," *Klinische Wochenschrift*, vol. 15, pp. 150–151, 1936.

H. Schnetz, "Vitamin C and Leucocyte Numbers," *Klinische Wochenschrift*, vol. 17, pp. 267–269, 1938.

12. P. Plum and S. Thomsen, "Remission in the Course of Aleukemic Leukemia," *Ugeskrift for Laeger* (Kobenhavn), vol. 98, pp. 1062–1067, 1936.

S. Heinild and Schiedt, "Remissions During Course of Leukemia Treated with Ascorbic Acid," *Ugeskrift for Laeger* (Kobenhavn), vol. 98, pp. 1135–1136, 1936.

W. Thiele, "Effect of Vitamin C on the White Blood Cells and Chronic Myeloid Leukemia," *Klinische Wochenschrift*, vol. 17, pp. 150–151, 1938.

C. L. C. van Nieuwenhuizen, "Effect of Vitamin C on the Blood Picture of Patient with Leukemia," *Nederlands Tijdschrift voor Geneeskunde* (Amsterdam), vol 7, pp. 896–902, 1943.

13. A. Vogt, "Vitamin C Treatment of Chronic Leukemias," *Deutsche Medizinische Wochenschrift,* vol. 66, pp. 369–372, 1940.

E. D. Kyhos et al., "Large Doses of Ascorbic Acid in Treatment of Vitamin C Deficiencies," *Archives of Internal Medicine,* vol. 75, pp. 407–412, 1945.

A. L. Waldo and R. E. Zipf, "Ascorbic Acid Level in Leukemia Patients," *Cancer,* vol. 8, pp. 187–190, 1955.

14. E. Greer, "Alcoholic Cirrhosis; Complicated by Polycythemia Vera and then Myelogenous Leukemia and Tolerance of Large Doses of Vitamin C," *Medical Times* (Manhasset), vol. 82, pp. 865–868, 1954.

III

Alternative Treatments

10

Charles Huggins on Hormone Therapy

I have many happy memories of the University of Chicago Clinics, where I interned in 1945. Things went very well. I spent the first three months happily delivering babies, then transferred over to Billings, where I was assigned to work under Dr. Charles Huggins, who was professor of urology and chairman of the department.

Dr. Huggins was then a young man of forty-four (he's now a vigorous seventy-seven). He was small, slender, and agile, and walked on his toes like a bantamweight boxer. He was one of the busiest men I have ever known. He did surgery in the mornings, attended to patients in the afternoon, and somehow found time to turn out the quality of research that won him a Nobel prize in 1966. Almost every honor imaginable has fallen Dr. Huggins's way.

I wrote him a letter, not one, but two. The first was addressed to his home and the second to his office at the university. (After thirty-three years you don't take chances.) After giving time for the letters to arrive, I telephoned his office, and who should answer but Dr. Huggins himself!

Sure, he would not only give me an interview but he'd buy the first copy of the book. I asked him to wait a moment while I switched on the tape recorder.

Then we had our chat.

INTERVIEW WITH DR. CHARLES HUGGINS

H. L. NEWBOLD: The first thing I would like to ask you is what percentage of patients with prostate cancer are helped by having female hormones administered to them?

C. HUGGINS: The figure has been for many years running around 80 percent. Approximately 80 percent of the men who receive estrogens [female sex hormones] show improvement in their condition.

HLN: Are we talking about a two- or three-year response?

CH: Two years and up.

HLN: Up to what?

CH: Indefinite. It may be anywhere from two years on up. They may have a remission lasting the rest of their natural life.

HLN: What percentage would you say have a long-term remission? By long-term I mean those that live out their natural life span.

CH: It's difficult to give the exact figures on those.

HLN: Well, I'm not talking about exact figures. I mean approximate figures. What would you say, 5 or 10 percent?

CH: I would put the number around 10 percent, if I had to make a guess.

HLN: Do you think every patient who has prostatic cancer should have his testicles removed?

CH: It is essential that every patient have an orchidectomy [removal of the testicles].

HLN: Do you think the operation should be done as soon as the diagnosis is made, or do you think that patients should have that done later, when the disease has progressed?

CH: The operation should be carried out as soon as the diagnosis of prostatic cancer is made. One hundred percent of the patients should have immediate orchidectomy.

HLN: Let me ask you what you think about X-ray therapy for cancer of the prostate.

CH: I think X-ray therapy to the prostate gland is a very valuable procedure and should be carried out in all patients if they do not have the prostate gland removed.

HLN: Do you feel that the cancerous prostate gland should be removed surgically?

CH: This is a very specialized type of surgery and requires considerable skill. However, if a surgeon skilled in this operation is available, I think the prostate gland should be removed. If the gland is not removed, then the patient should have X-ray therapy.

HLN: If the cancerous gland is removed by surgery, do you think the patient should still be given X-ray therapy?

CH: No, in that case then I don't think X-ray treatment should be given, but the patient should have an orchidectomy and should be given estrogen hormones.

HLN: What do you think of chemotherapy for the treatment of cancer of the prostate?

CH: I think chemotherapy is definitely not indicated for cancer of the.prostate. In general, I do not think that chemotherapy should be used for anything except for Hodgkin's disease, the lymphomas, and acute leukemias of childhood. I am very much opposed to chemotherapy as it is generally practiced. The iatrogenic * effect is tremendous. The patients feel worse with the chemotherapy than they do with the cancer.

HLN: It sounds as though you very much agree with a statistician I spoke with named Bross at the Roswell Park Memorial Cancer Institute in Buffalo.

CH: I am very much against chemotherapy, generally. It simply makes the patients too ill. Remember, there are worse things than death. One of them is chemotherapy.

HLN: What is your opinion about giving chemotherapy to women with breast cancer?

CH: It should not be given.

---

* When illness is produced by the treatment (in this case, by the use of chemotherapy).

HLN: Do you think women with breast cancer should be given testosterone [male sex hormone]?

CH: No, I don't think testosterone is indicated for that condition.

HLN: What about removing the ovaries? Do you think this should be done?

CH: In general, if a woman is less than fifty-three years old, I think her ovaries should be removed. Certainly her ovaries should be removed if she is still menstruating. Also, they should be removed if the woman stopped menstruating only two or three years ago. Bear in mind that the older a woman is when she is still menstruating, the more likely she is to develop breast cancer.

HLN: What do you think about birth control pills? Do you think they contribute to cancer of the breast?

CH: No, quite the contrary. I think that birth control pills, if anything, prevent women from developing breast cancer.

HLN: Do you have any thoughts about men taking testosterone? For example, many athletes and weight lifters use testosterone compounds in order to increase their physical abilities.

CH: No, I don't think that is a contributor to cancer of the prostate in men.

HLN: What do you think about natural resistance against cancer? Do you think there is such a thing?

CH: Yes, of course some people have more natural resistance against cancer than others. The disease tends to progress quicker in some individuals than others.

HLN: Do you think that nutrition has anything to do with this?

CH: No, I don't have any information about that or any reason to think that nutrition has a bearing on it.

HLN: Are you familiar with the work Linus Pauling and Ewan Cameron have been doing in Scotland, where they are treating cancer with vitamin C?

CH: Linus Pauling is a good friend of mine. I'm very fond of him.

HLN: Yes, I am aware of that. But what do you think about his advocating vitamin C to treat cancer?

CH: I think that's a lot of nonsense.

HLN: How familiar are you with the work he's done? Have you read the reprints about his work in Scotland?

CH: Linus is always mailing material to me.

HLN: Yes, but do you read it?

CH: Well, I glance through it.

HLN: What about the paper he did on his work involving 1,100 terminally ill cancer patients? He matched 100 treatment cases with a 1,000 control cases. The 100 patients he treated lived on an average four times as long as those he did not treat.

CH: Well, I just don't think vitamin C is effective against cancer. I've seen one patient who had vitamin C for cancer and it didn't help him. Of course, one patient doesn't mean anything.

I think we are only beginning to take the first steps toward understanding and treating cancer.

HLN: Anything else you would like to say to the general public?

CH: Men with prostatic cancer should have orchidectomies and should be given estrogen. At least 80 percent of them will have their lives significantly lengthened.

HLN: Thank you very much for your interesting interview.

CH: Let me know when the book comes out. I'll be the first to buy a copy of it.

HLN: I'll do better than that—I'll send you a free copy! Anything else to say to the public?

CH: Only that you're quite a guy.

HLN: Thank you very much. HLN (*to himself*): Now what does he mean by that?

11

The Case for Chemotherapy

Since a patient with cancer is often called upon to decide whether or not he wants chemotherapy, I have included both a pro-chemotherapy and an anti-chemotherapy chapter in this book in order to provide information that will be helpful in reaching a conclusion.

Mrs. Nay made one kind of decision, you will recall. Although vitamin C therapy can be given along with chemotherapy, sometimes a patient, such as Mrs. Nay, chooses between the two treatments.

Anyone making the choice needs all the facts. Since the doctor who states the case to the patient is not always entirely objective, patients need to know about other opinions also.

MEMORIAL SLOAN-KETTERING CANCER CENTER

You've all heard about the Memorial Sloan-Kettering Cancer Center in New York. When people like Hubert Humphrey and Happy Rockefeller get cancer, that's where they go for treatment. No one questions that it's the cancer Mecca of the world, in regard to both research and treatment.

In this country alone, thirty billion dollars are spent each year on cancer. When you walk in the front door of Memorial, you know at once where a good slice of that money goes. I couldn't help contrasting it to the Vale of Leven General Hospital, where Ewan Cameron does his work.

In the foyer at Memorial, you find a polished terazzo floor and pleasantly functional modern furniture. A guard stands near the doorway to give you directions. A bright young PR miss meets you and guides you up the smoothly functioning stainless-steel escalator, down the pleasant hallways to the pneumatic bliss of efficient elevators that lift you heavenward in the new skyscraper building.

Dr. Joseph Burchenal occupies a key position in the cancer complex as director of clinical research. In his eleventh-floor office, which commands a view of the Manhattan skyline, he looks very much like the general public's idea of a successful New York doctor: neatly dressed in a well-tailored suit, obviously bright, energetic, and sure of himself.

I hardly need add that he's pro-chemotherapy, as you will see from the chat we had.

Interview with Dr. Joseph Burchenal

H. L. Newbold: Dr. Burchenal, would you give us a thumbnail history of cancer chemotherapy? How long has it been around and how did it get started?

J. Burchenal: The first compound that had any effect on clinical cancer was a solution of potassium arsenite, which was given by Lissauer in 1886 to patients with chronic lymphocytic or chronic myelocytic leukemia. At about the same time, the famous surgeon Billroth used it for the treatment of lymphosarcoma and saw shrinkage of the tumor. From then on there was very little of this kind of treatment with chemotherapy, except for the sporadic use of benzol for chronic myelocytic leukemia in 1912 and 1921 by Kalapos and Koranyi, which did seem to produce remissions.

Potassium arsenite was studied again in the thirties by Claude Forkner and found to be definitely effective against CML [chronic myelocytic leukemia].

The effect of oophorectomy [removal of the ovaries] on carcinoma of the breast was first seen around 1890 by Bateman, and then further work was done on steroid hormones in the early forties. And, of course, Huggins did work on orchidectomy [removal of the testicles] for prostatic carcinoma in the 1940s.

HLN: Yes, I know about that. I was an intern on his service in 1945 when he was doing the work that later got him a Nobel prize.

JB: As far as regular chemotherapy is concerned, Haddow and his group tried urethane in the Walker 256 carcinoma and it did have activity. They tried it, along with Patterson and some others, for its effect against various types of solid tumors. But all they saw was leukopenia [a lowering of the total number of white blood cells], so then they tried it in chronic myelocytic leukemia. It did have a beneficial effect there, but it caused tremendous nausea and vomiting, very much the way arsenic had done. Then it was also tried by Rundles in multiple myeloma and thought to be useful.

Now we get to the nitrogen mustards. The mustards started with studies that were done after World War I, when two pathologists studied the bone marrows at autopsies on soldiers who had died of mustard gas poisoning and found that they were aplastic [not producing red and white blood cells].

That was published and forgotten about. I read it in 1940, but it really didn't click with me. Then, in 1942 or thereabouts, people were working on the nitrogen mustards and the sulfur mustards in the Chemical Warfare Service. They found that these chemicals did indeed cause atrophy of the spleen, lymph nodes, and bone marrow in animals. Then they tried it on an animal tumor. It caused an animal lymphosarcoma to shrink.

For that reason Goodman, Gilman, Lindskog, and Dougherty at Yale tried one of the nitrogen mustards, HN3, on a patient with lymphosarcoma. The great nodes in his neck and everywhere else shrank miraculously, but three weeks later they were back again.

They gave him a second dose and again the nodes decreased, but this time his bone marrow was hit pretty hard.* And I'm not sure whether they ever gave a third dose or not, but at any rate the disease slipped away from them. So then the alkylating agents came up from that. HN2 first. We tried a whole series of nitrogen mustards. We went on the assumption that if beta-chloroethyl groups were good, maybe four would be better. And we even got one that had eight such groups, but it didn't turn out to be any better. Haddow and his group got the idea that the alkylating groups were important but that it would be nice to have a carrier to get them to the right place, so they synthesized phenylalanine mustard, and since the L-phenylalanine was the physiologic isomer, they decided to try L-phenylalanine mustard. Elson felt there was a definite difference in the effectiveness of the L-pam versus D-pam.

While that was going on, Farber and Subba Row at Lederle were working on a folic acid antagonist. They had some very weak antagonists, the methyl folic and the folic with an aspartic acid instead of a glutamic acid. They thought these might be effective. And then they also had either a triglutamate or a heptaglutamate of folic acid. They were alleged by someone to be effective against animal tumors. Farber's story is that he tried these in patients and he had never seen the disease of acute leukemia exacerbated so much.

With that in mind, he asked Subba Row to make some strong antagonists. They knew the series of four amino antagonists where the hydroxyl in the 4 position of the pteridine ring was substituted by an amino group were very toxic agents. Aminopterin was the first one, and then it was followed by amethopterin, which was the 4 amino and N-10 methyl. Farber showed that he should get real remissions in children suffering from acute leukemia with aminopterin.

At approximately the same time, beginning in about

---

* The ability of the bone marrow to form red and white blood cells was almost knocked out.

1942, I believe, Heilman and Kendall, working at the Mayo Clinic, were studying compound E, a steroid, which turned out to be cortisone, and showed that in a single mouse with a lymphosarcoma almost the size of the mouse, this was able to make the tumor shrink down almost miraculously. But there was so little of the drug available that they couldn't do very many experiments. They delayed publication until about 1944 purposely because they knew there just wasn't any material available. When that finally came out, people got very interested in using it and ACTH [adrenocorticotropic hormone] on chronic lymphocytic leukemia and lymphosarcoma, and caused marked shrinkage of the nodes and tumors.

HLN: Why does that work, do you know?

JB: It's a lympholytic agent that works against the lymphoid tumor tissues but also works against normal immune mechanisms.

In 1949 the treatment of acute leukemia was enhanced by the use of cortisone or ACTH. So then we had steroids which could produce remissions very rapidly with relatively little toxicity, and aminopterin, which would produce remissions also. Then, in 1950, our group collaborating with Hitchings, and Elion at Burroughs Wellcome started working on diaminopurine, which supposedly was an adenine antagonist that produced an occasional remission in patients with acute leukemia, but really caused tremendous nausea and toxicity and was not worthwhile for any practical purposes. I used to say you had to have an iron man with copper-lined intestines to tolerate it. We did have one such patient with chronic myelocytic leukemia who had three consecutive remissions on the stuff, so there was no question but that it would cause remissions. We had one two-year remission, I think, in a patient with AML. But the real step forward was 6 mercaptopurine synthesized by Elion and Hitchings, which we first started working on clinically in 1952 and published on in 1953. That would produce remissions again in acute lymphoblastic leukemia in a fairly good percentage and occasionally in acute myelocytic leukemia in adults, maybe in about 10 percent of the patients. But it had the advantage that it would work in children whose disease was resistant to aminopterin. And so this added another class of drugs to our armamentarium. And of course since then many new drugs have been discovered.

HLN: Could you tell the general public briefly what is the theory behind chemotherapy?

JB: We want to find a drug which, when taken systematically by the patient, either by mouth or by injection, will seek out and kill the tumor cells at doses which are not toxic to the most sensitive normal cells. That's a big order, but it has been achieved in infectious diseases.

Penicillin, for instance, can be taken in large enough quantities to kill pneumococcus without being toxic to man. The sulfanilamides also work very well against the streptococcus. The streptococcus has a need, for instance, for para-amino benzoic acid as a nutrient, and the sulfanilamides are antagonists of this. Man had no need of para-amino benzoic acid. He could not use it at all, so therefore the sulfanilamides were essentially nontoxic to man. Now we don't have anything that's quite as black-and-white as that in chemotherapy. For instance, 6 mercaptopurine given to a child continuously on a day-to-day basis in the right dose will knock the leukemia cells down from 100 percent to 0 percent. The myeloid cells will come back up, the erythroid cells will come back up, and the platelets will come back up. If you give half of that dose, you probably won't make the leukemic cells come down. If you were to give twice that much you'd make the leukemic cells come down, but you'd inhibit the normal cells.

HLN: What percentage of patients experience toxic effects from chemotherapy?

JB: Well, it depends what the chemotherapy is. If you use prednisone, almost no one feels very bad. On the other hand, if you give cis-platinum I would guess almost 100 percent of them will have nausea and vomiting. But again you have to realize that the chemotherapy may have a chance of curing the patient against his almost sure death without it. Most patients are quite willing to take a little toxicity, a little discomfort. Also, for instance, many of these drugs make the hair come out, but this is temporary. The hair grows back as soon as you stop chemotherapy.

HLN: Why do they lose their hair?

JB: Well, apparently the hair follicle cells have much the same sensitivity to many of these agents that the cancer cells have, and the result is that when you give the chemotherapy to damage the cancer cells, you also damage the hair follicles. What happens is during the time that you have a high level of a particular drug in the body (which may be only twenty-four to forty-eight hours), the hair passing through the hair follicles, instead of coming out as a straight line, has a weakness in it, is much thinner. The result is that eventually, when the hair gets out beyond the hair follicles and then is brushed, it may well break off.

HLN: How long is chemotherapy administered? Is it given in courses or for the rest of the cancer patient's life?

JB: That depends on what your aim is. With acute leukemia in children, where you expect to cure the disease, you give it for two, two and a half to three years. Then you stop treatment. By that time at least 50 percent of the children will be cured of the disease. We are beginning to divide the acute leukemias in children into subtypes. It may be that as high as 80 or 90 percent of some of the subtypes will go on to long-term survival with proper care.

HLN: There was something in a newspaper in Boston recently about a mother who wanted her child to stop taking chemotherapy because she said the child felt so bad from it.

JB: Well, it depends on the drug. During the treatment of acute leukemia most of the children go to school and live their normal life. They may not feel quite up to snuff.

We had a guy who was on chemotherapy for his

acute leukemia for three years, during which time he made the freshman soccer team at the University of Connecticut. The next year he made the varsity, and the third year he was captain of the varsity and was on the all–New England team. He was on treatment pretty constantly. He'd come in here and he'd be so sick in between times that I would say "Good night, I'll see you in the morning" to him and I'd think the chances of my seeing him in the morning were pretty slim. But he'd be there in the morning, and a week or two later he'd be running ten blocks to get his strength back.

HLN: He had leukemia?

JB: Yes, he had leukemia. He was a guy that now, I'm reasonably sure, could be cured with the new drugs available. Unfortunately, his disease began a year or two too soon.

HLN: What neoplasms are treated most successfully with chemotherapy?

JB: Acute leukemia in children and Hodgkin's disease. I mean advanced Hodgkin's disease, because you would treat early Hodgkin's disease with radiation. Non-Hodgkin's lymphoma is doing much better, particularly in children. Wilms' tumor, with the combination of surgery, radiotherapy, and chemotherapy, has gone up to about 80 percent cure rate. Choriocarcinoma in the female is a good case in point. You've got 85 to 90 percent cure rate there. Combination therapy for testicular tumors in young men gives us a 50 percent long-term survival rate.

HLN: What do you mean by long-term?

JB: Well, you can't say exactly, because these new drugs have been in use only four or five years and they're constantly changing, made better. We've got patients with acute leukemia surviving 26 years and they don't show any signs of relapsing. In fact, I collected a series of acute leukemics about fifteen years ago. When I entered them in the books I put them down by the name of their doctors. This was very unfortunate, because some of these patients have outlived three doctors. It makes it somewhat difficult to find out just where they are.

HLN: What percentage of cancers would you say have highly satisfactory results with chemotherapy? Are we talking about 5 percent of all neoplasms or are we talking about 25 percent?

JB: That would be awfully hard to say. The hemotologic neoplasms [leukemias] are supposed to make up about 10 percent of all the cancers.

HLN: And they're the most successful?

JB: They're the most successful. But not all of them are responding well. The chronic granulocytic and chronic lymphocytic leukemias at the present time are doing about as well as they have been doing for the past twenty years. They do reasonably well on chemotherapy, but we haven't made any great strides. Certainly choriocarcinoma responds well, but that's a very rare tumor. Testicular tumors in young men are fairly common, but they make up a relatively small percentage of all tumors. We're doing a lot better than we used to with head and neck tumors, combining chemotherapy, surgery, and radiation. It looks as though oat cell carcinoma of the lung, which is an extremely malignant, very rapidly killing disease, and not at all amenable to surgery, may be controllable in 30 to 40 percent of the cases with aggressive chemotherapy. But these are early studies and it's too soon to say. That's going on the assumption that a certain percentage of those who are doing well with no evidence of disease at one or two years, whereas ordinarily the cancer kills in about three or four months, may possibly be cured. Burkitt's tumor, a tumor seen in Africa which is very common, has about a 50 to 60 percent cure rate, maybe higher in the early stages.

HLN: What total percentage are we talking about? Ten or 15 percent maybe?

JB: I would guess 15, maybe 20 percent, or something like that. It depends. It looks as though in premenopausal breast carcinoma, for instance, with positive nodes, chemotherapy is certainly delaying recurrence. Now, breast cancer is characteristically something which may come back in five, ten, fifteen, twenty years, so one still can't be sure whether it's a delay in development of recurrences or whether it's really a prevention of recurrences, but it's still holding up well.

The postmenopausal women with breast cancer aren't doing so well. We need better treatment there. With rectal cancer and most of the other cancers, chemotherapy tends to be palliative.

Diffuse histiocytic lymphoma in adults used to be a very rapidly growing tumor, very similar to oat cell carcinoma of the lung.* It killed very rapidly. It has been reported that maybe 40 to 50 percent of those may be curable, but you've got to go after it hard. Patients with this type of disease must be treated in centers that know how to treat it and are willing to be aggressive in treatment. This calls for courage on the part of both the doctor and the patient. With this type of disease you can kill more patients with kindness than you can with drugs, and if you say "Jim's such a nice guy we don't want to make him too sick, we don't want to make his hair fall out again or make him vomit too much," and so on, if you're a little easy with him, then the disease comes back and kills him.

HLN: When do you decide that this is all the chemotherapy a patient gets, that there's no point in pushing it any longer?

JB: When you run out of drugs that work. There are a certain number of drugs that are known, let's say, to be effective in Hodgkin's disease, and you try those and they don't work, and then, if you have some new drugs that look to be effective—say, they're effective in animal tumors and in tumors of a type that might predict for Hodgkin's disease—you might try those on the patient.

HLN: What if the patient was terminal, bedridden, not keeping food down, and so forth. When does one stop chemotherapy, if ever?

---

* This, you will recall, is the type of cancer Rosemary Nay has in Chapter 2.

JB: It depends what the disease is, to a large extent. For instance, if the patient has lung cancer and his bones are riddled with the disease, and you've tried your best treatment (there aren't many very good ones anyway) and the disease seems to be progressing, and he's obviously in a great deal of pain and all, I'd say there was no point in treating him further, if you had tried your best protocols. Sometimes you reach the stage where you give up.

HLN: How widespread in the United States is the relative sophisticated use of chemotherapy for neoplasms?

JB: Well, that depends. Different groups may have expertise in different areas. Take acute leukemia, for example. If you get a group of people who are interested in acute leukemia and they have all the new drugs and supportive hospital facilities where platelets are available and white cell transfusions and so on, then they can treat it very well. On the other hand, if the general internist or general pediatrician says, "Well, leukemia I can treat. I can treat them with a little prednisone and 6 mercaptopurine and maybe some vincristine. I won't make them sick," Johnny will go to school for a year and he'll be happy, and that's fine. But that ruins our chance of getting a combination which includes those drugs and several others that would have a good chance to cure him. That happens all too often.

HLN: If someone is in cardiac failure in Sioux City, Iowa, or in Idaho or Arizona, he is going to get digitalis and a salt-free diet and diuretics—in short, he's likely to get a good quality of help. How readily available is excellent chemotherapy for the country at large?

JB: There are quite a few co-operative groups. There's the Children's Cancer Group A. There's the Cancer and Acute Leukemia Group B, which has some thirty or forty different groups in it, and the Children's Cancer Group is equally big. There's the Eastern Cooperative Group (ECOG), and South-western Oncology Group. They're spread around so that most of the cities in the country have a group.

HLN: What percentage of people who should be treated with chemotherapy are being treated with it?

JB: I can't say for certain.

HLN: I understand you don't have exact figures, but if you were to guess at a figure, what would it be?

JB: Well, I would guess that at least 50 percent or maybe more are getting some type of chemotherapy. There are a lot of medical oncologists out in practice, and there are getting to be more and more all the time. This is an expanding field. It's expanding both in size and quality.

Remember, some of the new drugs and new combinations are essentially experimental. We don't know whether or not they're good. We think they're going to be better, but we don't know. For that reason, they're studied by co-operative groups at first until they demonstrate their excellence. And then they are able to get past the FDA and get sent out to the more general area.

HLN: Do they do double-blind studies on these?

JB: Not so much double-blind studies. It's too dangerous with chemotherapeutic agents that are toxic in themselves to do a double-blind. A randomized study, yes. Sometimes you do a double-blind study, but it's pretty hard. A good chemotherapist knows the drugs he's giving. He knows the toxic signs, so he wouldn't be far into the double-blind before he would know what he was giving. Personally, I wouldn't want to go into a double-blind study unless it was a question of a relatively nontoxic analgesic or something to keep a patient from vomiting. But these drugs differ so much in toxicity. For instance, BCNU or some of the nitrosoureas you give a single dose or two doses and then you wait and no leukopenia occurs for five or six weeks. On the other hand, with Cytoxan patients get their leukopenia in two weeks. If one were doing a double-blind study with one of the nitrosoureas at day 1 and then in two weeks there was no leukopenia, one might be tempted to give it again and again, and get into real trouble, so I wouldn't want to do it.

HLN: Which neoplasms are least successfully treated with chemotherapy?

JB: There are a lot of them vying for that honor. I think melanoma, when it gets beyond the skin. Cutaneous melanoma responds to lots of things, but visceral melanoma responds very poorly. Carcinoma of the lung responds rather poorly, if you leave out the oat cell carcinoma. Carcinoma of the colon responds a bit to 5-fluorouracil, but not too well. We're getting so many new agents now that it's hard to say. Head and neck tumors we used to think didn't respond very well, but with cis-platinum and bleomycin we're getting some quite good responses there, and even with esophageal cancers, cis-platinum and bleomycin seems to be doing surprisingly well.

HLN: It's too early to say for sure?

JB: That's right. With most of these new drugs and new combinations, it's too early to say. All you can say is you're getting some shrinkage. How long the shrinkage is going to last we don't know. Whether we're going to be able to continue giving the drugs and keep the tumor down; whether the tumor will get discouraged and go away; whether it will get to a point where the surgeon can take it out; or, if the surgeon has taken it out, whether the treatment is really preventing or just delaying its recurrence, we don't know.

HLN: Have you an opinion about reports of Ewan Cameron and Linus Pauling in their use of vitamin C to treat cancer?

JB: I haven't any scientific knowledge of that. I haven't heard of any evidence that it really is doing anything.

HLN: Are you familiar with the control study in Scotland where they used 100 treated patients and 1,000 controls?

JB: I have heard about it, but I've not gone into it in detail.

HLN: Do you do any nutritional support for patients who are getting chemotherapy?

JB: Yes, we use hyperalimentation * particularly for children with embryonal rhabdomyosarcoma † and lymphosarcoma when a tumor near the gut must be radiated. We're trying to keep the gut still and quiet.

HLN: What do you think about the concept Linus Pauling and others have about patients having resistance to cancer? We talk about resistance to flu and resistance to colds and so forth—what do you think about the conception of resistance to cancer? Many people are probably exposed to the cancer-producing agents or chemicals and so forth, and some people get cancer and some don't.

JB: I think that is a very definite factor. There must be a certain genetic susceptibility to cancer. Take as a case in point those individuals within a thousand meters of the hypocenter of the atomic bomb blast at Hiroshima. Among the survivors the incidence of leukemia went up, let's say, fifty-fold, so obviously heavy-dose radiation was extremely leukemogenic there. But, to look at the other side of the coin, only one out of fifty of those that were in that area and survived the explosion came down with leukemia. So if your genes are arranged right you get some protection. It's the same way with smokers. Smoking causes most lung cancer, but the converse is not that most smokers get lung cancer. Many of them don't.

HLN: Do you think that factors other then genetic . . .

JB: I think there is resistance to cancer because we know of a few anecdotal reports of patients who had pathologically proven cancer. Their abdomens were opened up, biopsied, and closed up, and then they were sent home to die. Then they happened to see the

---

* A type of artificial feeding involving the use of processed proteins, carbohydrates, and fats together with certain vitamins and minerals.

† Cancer that afflicts the muscles.

doctor ten years later and were perfectly healthy—without any treatment at all.

HLN: That's 1 in 100,000.

JB: Well, it's a very small percentage—something like that, I suppose. Then there are cases of what we call "unknown primaries," where a carcinoma or a melanoma metastasis develops, let's say in the lymph nodes. I have a patient like that right now. His first evidence of tumor was a swelling of the lymph nodes. Now, these particular types of tumors do not develop originally in the lymph nodes. They metastasize [spread] to the lymph nodes. But wherever that tumor was, presumably someplace on the back or on the chest or on the neck, it's gone. Nobody did anything to it. It wasn't biopsied. They never saw it. It went away itself. So that shows that the patient must have had some resistance against his tumor.

HLN: Do you think there's anything people can do to increase their resistance?

JB: A great deal of the anticancer effort is studying the immunologic reactivity of patients with cancer and trying to improve it with immunotherapy.

HLN: No, I'm not talking about that. I'm talking about something else. Mothers say, "Wrap up warm, honey, so you won't get pneumonia," or "Take your vitamins so you'll be healthy," or something. In your opinion, is there anything people can do to increase their natural resistance to cancer?

JB: If they could figure some way to keep under the age of forty that would be fine. As you age your immunologic reactivity is supposed to go down. Now whether there's anything that could somehow keep a seventy- or eighty-year-old man with the immunologic reactivity of the man of forty—I imagine there are people who have—why, that might be good. But I don't know what it would be. I suppose keeping in good health generally would be good.

HLN: It wouldn't be harmful, anyway.

JB: Yes, certainly you ought to try to keep yourself in good shape, although who was it, Clarence Demar, who used to run the Boston Marathon? He ran in marathons until he was sixty-nine or something like that, but he eventually died of cancer of the prostate, I think. So you can't tell. Of course, the obvious answer is that you've got to die sometime anyway. But there are certain things that probably cut down on your resistance. It may well be that many of these carcinogens just destroy your resistance. You know the theory of Sir McFarland Burnett, the surveillance theory, that says cells in our body are mutating constantly and every once in a while they throw off a neoplastic [cancer] cell. The body immediately recognizes it as "not self" and jumps on it and destroys it. And on the other hand, if you get a big dose of radiation or something which cuts down the body's immunologic capabilities, then these defenses wouldn't be able to destroy that cell and it might go on and grow into a tumor. And I suppose there are other things.

HLN: Like what?

JB: Well, I don't know what they would be, whether some of the carcinogens may be working that way or whether they're working more directly to cause a mutation. I don't think we know.

HLN: Do you think that nutrition has any bearing on this?

JB: The figures on the incidence of different types of cancer with different types of nutrition are interesting. For instance, Burkitt * says the diet in Africa has a very high fiber content, very low animal-fat content, and that they have almost no colon carcinomas or appendicitis or diverticulitis. Here in this country, we have low-fiber diets, a high animal-fat, and we have a high rate of colon carcinoma. In Japan they have a very low rate of breast cancer. Here we have a high rate of breast cancer. We eat much more fat.

HLN: Are you familiar with Dr. Schlegel's work? He is the professor and chairman of the department of urology at Tulane and uses vitamin C to prevent bladder cancer in smokers.

---

* D. P. Burkitt, the man who started the current interest in high-fiber diets.

JB: No, I'm not familiar with that. I do know of the theory that bladder cancer is one of the cancers that comes from smoking.

HLN: One of the criticisms about chemotherapy in patients in which it is marginally helpful is that it robs patients of the quality of their life.

JB: Well, you have to weigh everything. We have a case in point right now. Chronic myelocytic leukemia is a disease which characteristically goes on about three years. The patient can be maintained in good health with Myleran therapy and he does extremely well. This time may be plus or minus a year or so. I just had one patient who lived ten years. At the end of that time he went into an acute exacerbation for which we have no treatment and went downhill and died in a month or less. There hasn't been any improvement in treatment for chronic myelocytic leukemia in twenty-five years, or maybe even longer. We have recently tried a new form of treatment in which we treat those patients aggressively, as if they had acute leukemia. We had one moderately aggressive regimen which frequently seemed to decrease the number of pH-positive cells. And the ones where we did succeed in decreasing the pH-positive cells, or getting them down to zero, are doing better so far as their longevity is concerned. They seem to do better than the patients who were previously treated with Myleran. Now we've developed an even more aggressive form of treatment. I can speak feelingly about it because I have a patient on it right now and I have talked to him many times about it. This patient was given a choice of three years of good, perfectly normal life with no hospitalization or our new aggressive treatment, for which he would need to come into the hospital for four or five days every three weeks. This would amount to approximately three months of hospitalization during the first year. And after that, presumably, no hospitalization but chemotherapy as an outpatient for another two years. He might be cured but also might not be.

After discussing this treatment in great detail, a

certain number of patients have opted for this and a lot of others have opted against it.

HLN: What are your feelings? Do you think that this is just an individual thing?

JB: I think each person has to make the decision. If they want to take our aggressive treatment, I think there is a chance that it might work out. I just honestly don't know. If this were a situation where I knew we could cure a certain percentage it would be different, but we don't know.

HLN: What would you do if you had chronic myelocytic leukemia?

JB: I think that under the circumstances I would tend to opt for the aggressive treatment, but I may be optimistic.

HLN: So generally you think the patient simply has to decide what horse he's going to bet on, and act accordingly.

JB: That's right. The patient must give informed consent on all these cases, and you have to discuss it in detail in all its ramifications. For instance, a patient who knows all about cancer and is an extremely knowledgeable person and knows that probably she ought to get chemotherapy may not take it because it interferes with her job and makes her feel too sick.

The myth of immortality is also a problem. Patients say, "Well I know that 80 percent of the patients with four positive nodes in the axilla are going to be dead at the end of ten years, but 20 percent of them are going to be living. I'm going to be in that 20 percent, so I won't bother to take the treatment."

That's why smokers don't stop smoking when the doctors say, "You've got a high risk of getting cancer of the lung because you smoke three packs a day." Many will just say, "I'll take my chances." But if they start to get symptoms of Buerger's disease * and their feet start tingling and so forth, and the doctor says, "Okay, you stop smoking or you stop skiing, maybe

---

* A closing up of arteries, often caused by smoking tobacco. —H.L.N.

even stop walking," they never have another cigarette. So it is up to the patient to make up his or her mind. What you try to do is to give them the facts.

I have a patient now with oat cell carcinoma we are treating and we have made him pretty darn sick at intervals over a period of two years. But the usual survival time in this disease is about four months, and he's got no evidence of disease at the present time. He's now on the last cycle of treatment. Hopefully, he'll be free of disease.

HLN: The problem is this: Since vitamin C, ascorbic acid, is a strong detoxifier, would it protect the patient's cancer cells as well as the normal cells against chemotherapy?

JB: I have no idea about that.

HLN: Are there any final words that you would like to give the general public about chemotherapy for cancer?

JB: Yes, I think the important thing to say is that there are a lot of advances being made in chemotherapy. By advances I mean really going from the side of palliative to curative therapy. It takes these techniques a certain time to percolate down from the people who discover them to the general practitioner and the general public. So I think it's terribly important that patients with acute leukemia, Hodgkin's disease, lymphomas, or with testicular, ovarian, or oat cell carcinoma be referred as soon as possible to a center that is specializing in that sort of disease. They should not be treated first and then sent in. For instance, in acute leukemia in children, what the pediatrician who makes the diagnosis does is extremely important. The important thing for him to do is to send the child to a center. He and the center can then plan together on a course of treatment for this child for the next three years. The patient will then return to the pediatrician, who will be responsible for the treatment. Maybe the child will return to the center once a month, or something like that, for a checkup.

What the diagnosing pediatrician does is extremely important. He can't do it alone. He doesn't have all the newest drugs. He doesn't have the latest know-how. It may be that what he thinks is very good was top-notch stuff five years ago—but we've made a lot of progress since then.

We're constantly trying to keep up with what's going on. Somebody in Paris may find a drug that's red-hot. We try to keep in constant contact, because we don't want our patients to die for lack of a drug which is available that we don't happen to know about. That's why ever since we've been in this business many of us have tried to keep on a first-name basis with investigators in Paris, in London, in Milan, in Moscow, and in Japan—all over, so that whenever anything new comes along we can let each other know about it in a hurry. We've always done that.

The important thing is to get the patient at a time when chemotherapy can do the most good.

Surgery will cure any cancer, no matter how big it is, so long as it's localized (providing you can take it out without removing a vital organ). But if it's widespread the surgeon can do little. Chemotherapy, on the other hand, will seek out tumors no matter where they are, but it's limited by the bulk of the tumor. If there's a lot of bulk, it's very hard for chemotherapy to cure it. With small tumors we've got much more chance of cure. That's why adjuvant chemotherapy with surgery and/or radiation is so important, because the other modalities reduce the bulk of the tumor and chemotherapy can penetrate the whole body and search out and kill the few remaining cancer cells. Thus, I think it's vital that these patients get to a center where the best treatment can be given just as soon as is humanly possible.

12

The Case Against Chemotherapy

I admire Irwin Bross. He stands up and speaks the truth as he sees it. If his views happen to upset a few billion-dollar apple carts, well, that's just too bad. Like me, he's a maverick who's forever throwing a handful of sand into the well-oiled machinery of the Medical Establishment.

Irwin D. J. Bross, Ph.D., is a biostatistician, a man whose full-time job is to help scientists plan valid research projects. He also analyzes research reports to decide whether their claims stand up from a statistical viewpoint.

The field of biostatistics is highly technical and specialized. Scientists stand somewhat in awe of this mathematical specialty and are generally ill at ease in its presence.

Every endeavor of mankind is open to criticism, whether it's the way a bridge is built or how a scientific experiment is set up. The mathematician is the man who is most likely to give the final appraisal.

Chemotherapists and radiologists are, as a group, not very fond of Dr. Bross, because he keeps telling them that their headway against treating cancer is negligible, with three exceptions: acute leukemia in children, the lymphomas, and early breast cancer.

He thinks chemotherapy for other types of cancer,

once it has spread, is largely a waste of time, that it simply makes the patient ill and doesn't significantly lengthen life. Chemotherapy is usually a mercenary placebo—a placebo more for the doctor than for the patient.

One of the problems is money. The public relations departments of almost every group engaged in fighting cancer like to give out optimistic reports. This steady flow of positive news keeps the flame of hope burning and keeps the dollars rolling in.

If the PR people said: "We're very discouraged about our search for a cause and treatment of cancer . . . We don't know what causes it and we don't know how to treat it . . . The problem seems almost hopeless," then the flow of money would stop.

And if the money stopped coming in, the directors of the societies, the public relations officers, and the secretaries would be out of work. The technicians and scientists would find their labs closed and themselves hat in hand, seeking a new job.

Looking at it from this standpoint, can you blame them for putting out favorable reports?

Can you understand why they don't like a maverick like Dr. Bross?

Dr. Bross has been in his field a long time. Originally he was at the Memorial Sloan-Kettering Cancer Center in New York, but he is now with a highly respected state institution in Buffalo, New York, the Roswell Park Memorial Institute for Cancer Research.

INTERVIEW WITH IRWIN BROSS

H. L. NEWBOLD: I would like to start by asking about the over-all progress in cancer chemotherapy in the last twenty-five years.

I. BROSS: I started at Memorial Sloan-Kettering about twenty-five years ago. That time was really the beginning of the present push toward chemotherapy. They were very enthusiastic. At that time, I too was somewhat caught up in the enthusiasm. The end results of chemotherapy after twenty-five years have been a disappointment for me. There has been some progress, but not much.

About twenty-five years ago they had a meeting on mercaptopurine for the treatment of childhood leukemia. At that time the eight or ten doctors who had used the drug reported transient remissions. We tried to discuss the results. They ended up asking me to put the data together. I studied the figures and information and decided to take a stand which was not expected.

I went back and told them they would never be able to get good answers if they only treated a couple of patients this way. Everybody used a different system of treatment. The only way to get good figures was to use controlled clinical trials. I had been working with the father of controlled clinical trials at Cornell at that time, the clinical pharmacologist Dr. Harry Gold.

To my surprise, to everybody's surprise, my recommendation was quite enthusiastically received. Out of this came the first clinically controlled trial in the United States of a collaborative kind. Dr. Burchenal was the leader. Well, as you know, this line of endeavor has produced substantial improvement in the treatment of childhood leukemia.

HLN: That is acute leukemia?

IB: Acute leukemia in children, ALL [acute lymphocytic leukemia]. It is a very rare child with leukemia that is not in that group. Research was very discouraging until perhaps the last ten years, when we began to have real improvements. Now people are starting to look at the problem. In the early days they had just been playing games with very minor things in the therapy; trying a new drug, trying this, that and the other without really attempting to learn from their failures. I'm an advocate of controlled clinical trials if people use them intelligently. I think the most adequate data on treatment results come from such trials.

HLN: Are there many controlled studies using chemotherapy against cancer?

IB: There are a large number, but many of them are not very good ones. They are not well controlled. Let's put it that way. The ALBG * trials were among the best. Actually, I think the controlled studies on leukemia that I helped set up (I hope you don't think I'm bragging) are among the best of their kind.

HLN: I think most people agree with that.

IB: And I've heard about a great many other trials. Sometimes they are well done, but many have been more or less nonproductive. And the other point I would get to on that is why so many of these trials end in failure. The treatment of solid tumors † with chemotherapy is pretty much a failure.

We are beginning to understand solid tumors better. I presented a paper on the subject in Washington on the eighth of April. I talked about the cascade process of metastasis. We have identified a sequence of events in the metastatic process. The tumor usually does not metastasize [spread] from the primary. It metastasizes from a metastasis. Sometimes the sequence is primary to lung and then generalized, and sometimes the sequence is primary to the liver and then lung, then generalized. Sometimes it is more complicated, like primary to bone to liver to lungs, but in every case it is quite a rigid sequence and we know the sequence.

Now, the main point is that once the tumor has generalized—that is to say, once it has spread to one of the metastatic sites—the site will generalize the tumor. At that point it really doesn't do a bit of good to treat the primary site with any expectation of cure. The primary is not the problem any longer. All this has been worked out using thousands of cases of autopsy material.

The main point is that if you try to go in with any

---

* The name for the specific group of doctors engaged in research.

† Solid tumors refers to forms of cancer other than leukemia.

form of treatment (including chemotherapy) after the spread of the cancer has occurred, you aren't going to cure the patient with anything we have now. That's where it stands.

As you know, the solid tumors are the kind of tumors they try to treat, but they fail, except for lymphomas and occasionally breast cancer. We were the first people to find results with almost homeopathic [minute] doses of thiotepa for breast cancer. That is where it stands, then: If you can get in on any of the cancers early enough, you have some fighting chance of curing the patient, but if you don't . . .

HLN: By early enough you mean before the metastasis?

IB: Before the cancer spreads from the original site to the generalizing site. This is a very simple point: You can almost say that if it hasn't gotten to the lungs, you have a chance. If it's gotten there, you don't have a chance with anything we have now. That doesn't apply to the leukemias or the lymphomas. All our studies have, I think, been on patients given chemotherapy as adjunct to surgery and radiation. Most of the patients receiving chemotherapy were not helped. Nothing could be expected to happen.

I wrote an article on this concerning breast cancer. We've developed a mathematical model for breast cancer. It's very easy to show that you really can't expect much if you treat breast cancer after it's metastasized. Then you are no longer treating breast cancer. You are treating a generalized disease. This is, in a nutshell, my position on the treatment of cancer. I think there has not been any substantial progress, any progress at all, in the treatment of the generalized disease.

HLN: Other than acute childhood leukemia and the lymphomas.

IB: They are the exceptions.

HLN: What would you do if you had cancer?

IB: It would depend on the stage. If I had metastasis I would try to live the rest of my life as peacefully and comfortably as I could.

HLN: Without chemotherapy?

IB: Without anything.

HLN: What if you had an oat cell carcinoma of the lung?

IB: No one can say in advance, before it happens, what he would really do. It could be different at the time. At this point, I would not be inclined to undergo surgery.

HLN: And you would forgo chemotherapy?

IB: Yes.

HLN: In view of the fact that chemotherapy usually makes patients quite ill, do you feel there is something immoral about treating patients with generalized cancer and making them miserable for the last months of their lives?

IB: I'm not loved by radiologists and chemotherapists. I don't think that we should be spending thirty billion dollars a year for the treatment of cancer. That's an enormous amount of money. Even with thirty billion a year we can't give patients much for their money. I think that there are places where even a billion dollars invested intelligently can be a benefit to a lot more people than spending it on people who are sixty-five or seventy or seventy-five, who are obviously going to die in two months or six months after a very unpleasant period.

I don't believe that it is the job of a physician to prolong the agony of a patient. This doesn't make me popular. I am not impressed with the palliative results that make these people live three months longer, on the average. They should either cure cancer patients or come close to it. Just dragging a life on for a few months is pointless. All the proponents of chemotherapy in the medical profession tell me that patients want a few more months, that this is what they demand.

When I talk to people who have cancer or to the relatives of cancer patients, this is not their attitude. They are not looking for the latest and greatest technology to be tried on these individuals. They are looking for something to cure them. If they can't be cured, the idea of keeping them under morphine for a

133

few months does not appeal to the patient, the family, or the public. I think you see this difference between the doctor's opinion of the public opinion and the true public opinion. Who wants the life-support systems being used to keep vegetables alive?

HLN: Would you have X-ray or cobalt treatments if you had cancer?

IB: If I was advised to take radiation I would know at that point I was terminal. I wouldn't bother.

HLN: I want this book to help people decide what treatment they want. I have the feeling that oncologists are giving patients pictures of chemotherapy that are unrealistically optimistic. Then they leave it up to the patient to decide about chemotherapy. That's why your viewpoint is so valuable for this book.

IB: I hope that more patients are getting a choice and take advantage of the choice. This has really been the whole business of Laetrile. It is not so much a drug issue. Many of the people who are involved in Laetrile are not actually patients, but it's a question of freedom of choice.

Your book should point out that the public wants the right to make vital choices, even on the question of dying.

HLN: I think that's a very important point.

IB: Because of the exposure of X rays, I've been opposed to mass-screening mammography. The women should have been given the information about the hazards of radiation at the same time they were given the sales talk for mammography. If they decided they wanted it, it would be their option. But they were never given the choice.

HLN: In other words, you would like to fully inform the general public?

IB: I think it's very confusing for the public to keep getting newspaper accounts of breakthroughs in cancer treatment. Biostatistics simply don't show that much improvement. When I testified on the mismanagement of the National Cancer Institute's program, I criticized their statistics. There has not been anything terribly optimistic to report except in a few cases. The one other thing I would say is that it is better to prevent cancer than to try to cure it. That has been my number one target.

HLN: In what direction do you think the general public should be led in preventing cancer?

IB: Well, I think basically most of the things that produce cancer are things that we've introduced in the past sixty to one hundred years: chemicals and radiation. The hard part about technology is using it intelligently. That's where we've broken down. Technology of itself is neither good nor bad.

HLN: Can you give me an example?

IB: I think the mass screening with mammography is a good example. Here you had a technology. Doctors were gung-ho to use it on a huge scale. They went right ahead and X-rayed not just a few women but a quarter of a million women. That use of technology was very foolish. A jump to the exposure of a quarter of a million persons to something which could do them more harm than good was criminal—and it was supported by money from the federal government and the American Cancer Society.

This is what I mean by a mindless way of using technology. One trouble with technology is the advocates always want to do things on a larger scale. If it hasn't worked on a limited scale, they always say, "Well, we'll use it on a bigger scale." But it never works out when used that way.

There hasn't been a big advance in chemotherapy, but I think saying everything is completely negative takes away hope, and that's not really my purpose. I just do not want to give any false hopes.

HLN: You mentioned thirty billion dollars. Do you mean that amount has been spent on cancer over a period of twenty-five years?

IB: I mean over one year.

HLN: Thirty billion?

IB: We spend 188 billion a year in the health industry.

HLN: Thirty billion, including what the patients spend?

IB: Government, patient, research, everything combined. Cancer is not the commonest disease, but it certainly is the most expensive. Cancer research costs the government something like 815 million dollars a year. If you made it a billion dollars you'd have all the research that is being done on cancer in this country, so that that's not a very great part of the billion.

HLN: Now, you deal in biostatistics—what is your exact title?

IB: I am Director of Biostatistics at Roswell Park Memorial Institute for Cancer Research. It's a state institution.

HLN: I'm very grateful for the interview, because it gives a valuable side to the cancer problem, one that people need to know. I think my book would have been very uneven if I hadn't interviewed you.

Once you get interested in a subject, information seems to flow your way, sometimes from the most unexpected quarters. I talked with Dr. Glenn Dettman in Australia one night about a new vitamin C product he is developing for intravenous treatment. A few days later he sent me a number of reprints, including an Australian Associated Press article that appeared in the Melbourne *Herald* on March 8, 1975, about James Watson's views on cancer research.

Many of you know James Dewey Watson as the man who received a Nobel prize for medicine in 1962 for his work at Cambridge University in unraveling the mystery of the DNA double helix.

Often, because of his work at Cambridge, he is thought to be English. Actually, he was born in Chicago. He was an undergraduate at the University of Chicago when I was interning there.

He was, as the article mentions, professor of molecular biology at Harvard. Since then, he has moved to suburban Long Island, and is now director of the Cold Spring Harbor Laboratory. He even looks suburban: paunchy with a round face and black hornrimmed glasses and a hairline that's beginning to recede out of sight.

Following is the Melbourne *Herald* AAP story. As you will see, he's not very favorably impressed with the quality of cancer research. Since he's a member of the American Association for Cancer Research, he must keep in touch with the subject.

AMERICA'S CANCER PROGRAM IS A SHAM,
ACCORDING TO NOBEL PRIZE–WINNING
BIOLOGIST JAMES WATSON

Despite millions of dollars being spent on rapid development of cancer treatment centres, the result may only be a facade with little increase in understanding cancer or knowing how to treat it, he said.

Dr. Watson, a professor of molecular biology at Harvard, spoke at a symposium on cancer research at the Massachusetts Institute of Technology.

"The American public is being sold a nasty bill of goods about cancer. While they're being told about cancer cures, the cure rate has improved only about one percent."

"The grim cancer statistics are about as bad as ever. Today, the press releases coming out of the National Cancer Institute have all the honesty of the Pentagon's."

Dr. Watson said a key problem was that the nation's best universities had failed to come up with major plans for attacking cancer.

In 1962, Dr. Watson shared the Nobel prize for medicine for his part in deciphering the molecular structure key to genetics.

That discovery is basic to much modern cancer and other research.

He criticised the $438 million national cancer plan, calling it "a total sham."

He questioned the effectiveness of the 16 institutions in the U.S. set up as comprehensive cancer centres. . . .

Another voice recently spoke out against the quality of research in the field of medicine. In the *Internal*

Medicine News, July 1, 1978, Dr. Thomas Chalmers, President and Dean of Mount Sinai School of Medicine in New York, was quoted as saying that only one third of the randomized, controlled studies which he investigated were well done. None of the randomized, controlled therapeutic studies reported in the *New England Journal of Medicine* or in *Lancet* during 1975 and 1976 was of excellent quality.

Which medical specialty ranked the lowest in quality of research? Cancer.

13

Seymour Levitt for Radiology

In 1948, when I finished my residence training in internal medicine, I went to a little town in North Carolina called Newton, where my salary was a princely $10,000 a year. I was employed strictly to practice internal medicine; however, several of the local general practioners liked to have a full day a week away from their practices, and a few others really didn't like getting up in the middle of the night. As a result, they made me an offer that would increase my income: If I would deliver babies for them on their days off or in the middle of the night, they would pay me twenty-five dollars in hard, immediate cash for doing each delivery.

I was glad to have the extra work delivering babies. During my internship at the University of Chicago I had had considerable experience in the field. As a matter of fact, it soon became apparent to the local doctors that I knew more about obstetrics than they did. They even started referring complicated delivery problems to me. I turned out to be a twenty-five-dollar bargain.

At any rate, I began to get more and more fascinated by the subject of obstetrics, and finally decided I wanted some more training in the field. A local businessman very generously loaned me the money I would need to get started, and I selected the University of Minnesota, where, in the winter of 1949, I began my second internship, this time in straight obstetrics and gynecology.

Although my interest was mainly in obstetrics, I spent nine months of that year in gynecology. The chief of service was Dr. John, McKelvey, who was very involved in cancer research, especially cancer of the uterus and cervix. As a result, I got a great deal of clinical experience with cancer. I helped in establishing the diagnosis, in charting the stage of cancer, and in the treatment, mainly surgery, X ray, and radium.

When I decided to have a chapter in the book on X-ray therapy, it was only natural that I should think of the University of Minnesota Medical School. Since my days there, the good taxpayers of the state have paid for more modern buildings that have expanded the already excellent medical center, which, as for many years, is tied closely to another well-known center, the Mayo Clinic at Rochester, Minnesota.

Here's my chat with Dr. Seymour Levitt, Professor of Therapeutic Radiology and chairman of the department at the University of Minnesota School of Medicine.

INTERVIEW WITH DR. SEYMOUR LEVITT

H. L. NEWBOLD: What forms of cancer do you feel are best treated with radiation therapy? What kind of results can you get?

S. LEVITT: First you must realize that radiation therapy can be used either alone or in a combination with surgery or with some type of chemotherapy.

Radiation alone is usually the treatment of choice for early head and neck cancer or early cancer of the oral cavity or of the vocal chords. With stage 1 cancer we're getting a 90 percent cure rate. In stage 2 cancer we're realizing about a 70 percent cure rate. These patients (not having had surgery) are able to maintain their voice and their tongue. They maintain their ability to speak and function and have as good a chance for cure as patients treated with surgery.

HLN: Are you talking about a five-year cure rate?

SL: Yes, a five-year cure rate.

Now I want to point out even with those patients in whom radiation is not successful, the patient still has the opportunity for surgery and eventual cure, what we call salvage surgery. Approximately 50 percent of cases where radiation fails can still be operated upon and have an excellent chance for cure.

HLN: What about skin cancer?

SL: With skin cancers, whether you're talking about the squamous cell or the basal cell type, we get a 90 to 95 percent cure rate with radiation therapy alone if we treat before there is metastasis [spreading].*

HLN: Do you still feel that radiation is the treatment of choice for skin cancers?

SL: I feel that radiation is the treatment of choice for most cancers of the skin, other than the melanomas. I think there are some instances—an older patient with a small lesion on the cheek, for example, or some area like that—when it is much quicker to operate and cut it out.

On the other hand, with cancer of the eyelid, ear, nose, or areas like that, where surgical excision would require plastic surgery later, the results with radiation therapy alone are equivalent to those of surgery. But with radiation therapy you avoid the necessity of plastic surgery later and the disability that goes with surgical procedures.

I think most ophthalmologic surgeons would agree that in eyelid cancer there's no question but that radiation therapy is the treatment of choice. It avoids the necessity for later reconstructive surgery.

HLN: Are large doses of radiation needed to treat skin cancers?

SL: No, no. Most patients, if they're treated properly, will have hardly any noticeable change in the appearance of the skin. This is particularly important in treating eyelids. Also, it is very important in younger

---

* The squamous cell carcinoma of the skin is the only one that metastasizes.

people. I think radiation therapy is certainly as good as, and in many instances superior to, surgery.

HLN: With what other cancers do radiation therapists get excellent results?

SL: In gynecologic cancer, of course. In most institutions in this country and in Europe, radiation therapy is the treatment of choice for cancer of the cervix.

HLN: John McKelvey was a great leader in that field there at the University of Minnesota, wasn't he?

SL: Yes, he was very prominent and influential in the field. The result is that in this institution, and in other leading institutions where radiation therapy has been used as the primary treatment for cancer of the cervix, our cure rates are as good if not better than the surgeon's, and we avoid a number of complications that can develop with surgery. We think radiation is the treatment of choice.

HLN: What about uterine cancer?

SL: Radiation can be used for uterine cancer, but for cancer of the body of the uterus radiation is almost always used in conjunction with surgery, except in those patients who are not operable because of serious medical illnesses.

HLN: What about cancer of the vulva [the external female genitalia]?

SL: Cancer of the vulva is usually treated with a combination of surgery and radiation therapy, but that is more of a surgical problem.

HLN: What percentage of cures are you talking about with cancer of the cervix?

SL: In stage 1 we get a 90 to 95 percent cure. Stage 2 goes down to about 75 to 80 percent. I'm talking about a five-year cure rate.

Radiation therapy is the treatment of choice for vaginal cancers in many institutions, including our own, places like M.D. Anderson, and in many European centers. This is a more difficult type of cancer to control. But we're getting about 70 to 75 percent cure rate in early cancer of the vagina.

Patients with seminomas of the testicle can be certain

of the 90 to 95 percent cure rate if both the surgery and radiation are in early use.

Incidentally, there is a tumor of the ovary in females called dysgerminoma which is extremely sensitive to radiation. Radiation in combination with surgery gives a high rate of cure when the cancer is detected early.

With Hodgkin's disease, radiation is the treatment of choice in stages 1 and 2.

This is a remarkable breakthrough for radiation therapy. When I was going to medical school Hodgkin's disease was considered incurable and hopeless. Now we're talking about an 80 to 95 percent cure rate in stage 1 with radiation alone, and 70 to 75 percent in stage 2. And remember, patients who fail radiation therapy can often be controlled by chemotherapy.

HLN: And your results with lymphomas are about the same?

SL: The difference with lymphomas has been that most patients are more advanced when seen initially. Stage 1 and stage 2 lymphomas have done very well with radiation therapy alone. One of the most malignant of the non-Hodgkin's lymphoma is called histiocytic lymphoma. We have treated a small group of stage 1's and have a 100 percent five-year survival rate.

HLN: How many patients?

SL: We're talking about 10 patients.

HLN: That's significant.

SL: We feel very encouraged by this.

HLN: Okay, what are your other best results?

SL: If you want to consider radiation therapy in conjunction with surgery, we should mention salivary gland tumors. Radiation therapy can improve the survival rate by 10 or 15 percent.

HLN: You can increase that percentage 10 or 15 percent?

SL: Right, and this is also true with carcinoma of the endometrium [lining of the uterus], where in early lesions radiation therapy is useful, particularly for more undifferentiated tumors and larger tumors. We improve the cure rate by 10 to 15 percent when radiation therapy is added to surgery.

HLN: How about prostate?

SL: In prostate—thank you for reminding me—that's an area where radiation alone has been extremely beneficial. We feel that it is the treatment of choice. In carcinoma of the prostate we are reporting five-year and even ten-year survivals, which are equivalent to surgical survival rates. In early lesions, we get somewhere between 60 and 70 percent five-year cures. That is certainly equivalent to what surgeons are reporting. One of the problems with carcinoma of the prostate is that it is an unpredictable disease. We have to wait between ten and fifteen years to be sure we have really cured the disease. But the experience at our center, and at the other larger centers like Stanford, where they have treated prostate cancer with radiation, shows survival rates equal to those of surgery without the side effects of surgery.

HLN: By side effects you mean impotence and inability to control the urinary stream and so forth?

SL: Right. Some patients have had a problem with impotence following radiation, but the incidence is far less than that following surgery. Incontinence [inability to control the urinary stream] has not been a problem with radiation therapy.

HLN: Do you advise removal of the testicles for cancer of the prostate?

SL: We do not.

HLN: If there's a progression of the cancer?

SL: There's really not been any evidence to demonstrate orchidectomy [removal of the prostate] adds to radiation therapy alone. Not initially, anyway. We prefer to wait. If the cancer progresses, that's another problem. But a number of published papers state that orchidectomy does not really add anything to the survival rate for patients treated with radiation.

HLN: And you don't give female sex hormones either for prostatic cancer?

SL: No. Only radiation therapy.

HLN: And what about breast cancers?

SL: Well, that is another controversial area, but we feel (and a number of my modern colleagues agree) that radiation therapy can be extremely useful in the treatment of early breast cancers combined with minimal surgery or local excision. There have been many recorded experiences in the medical literature of using simple local removal of small breast cancers (4 centimeters or less) and then treating with radiation. With stages 1 and 2, breast cancer patients had the same survival as those patients treated with radical mastectomy alone.

HLN: That's with local removal of the small breast cancer, followed by radiation?

SL: That's correct.

HLN: What survival rates are you talking about with breast cancer?

SL: We're talking about five-year survival rates of 80 to 90 percent with stage 1 cancers.

HLN: And if it's spread to lymph nodes?

SL: Well, we're talking about 60 to 65 percent five-year survival in stage 2 breast cancer.

HLN: Here again, as with cancer of the prostate, figures are difficult to come by.

SL: Breast cancer is a very unpredictable disease, and one has to follow a case for a long time to be sure. But our five-year cures are indicative (when compared with five-year cure rates with radical mastectomy) that we are on the right track. Our experience, as well as others', indicates that we are moving in the right direction and that our results are quite as good as with surgery alone, and the patient retains her breast with excellent cosmetic results in most cases.

HLN: Now, what group do you want to put next?

SL: One of the most interesting areas has been the treatment of soft tissue sarcomas with radiation therapy combined with minimal surgery. This success has been reported from a number of institutions. The cure rate has been really phenomenal. The local recurrence rate and the survival rate have been an equivalent to those for radical surgery. Of course, by radical surgery we mean amputation of an arm or a leg for this type of sarcoma. With radiation and minimal surgery, patients have preservation of limb and limb function, and a cure rate equivalent to that of radical surgery.

Then there's preoperative and postoperative radiation therapy in the treatment of bladder and rectal cancer. There has been a significant improvement in survival in the Duke's stage C rectal cancer, improving survival from around 35 percent for surgery alone to 50 percent when combined with radiation.

HLN: What kind of rectal cancer is that?

SL: That's C, the rectal cancer in which there is lymphatic metastasis. Also in bladder cancer, in the more advanced cases, patients treated with radiation plus surgery have a significant improvement in survival as compared to similar patients treated with surgery alone.

Incidentally, speaking about long-term effects, there are areas in childhood cancer where youngsters have been treated with radiation therapy following surgery with excellent results, whereas surgery alone gave dismal results. One of them is the medullablastoma, which is a brain tumor seen in children. With surgery alone there are virtually no survivers. But with surgery and radiation we have reported approximately a 70 percent survival rate with good function. And there's a role for radiation in Wilms' tumor, and in a number of other instances of childhood tumors.

HLN: With which types of cancer does radiation therapy give the poorest results?

SL: So far as cure rate is concerned, radiation therapy has really not been too effective in pancreatic tumors or gastric tumors and liver tumors. Melanomas have not been too effectively treated. Of course, the results in the more malignant brain tumors are very poor whatever agent is used.

HLN: And what about colon and lung cancers?

SL: Radiation therapy is effective as a palliative agent. But insofar as cure is concerned, we don't do too well with colon, rectal, and lung cancers. Although there have been some very encouraging results in early rectal cancer with radiation alone.

HLN: But in advanced colon cancer radiation may help by relieving obstructions.

SL: Yes, that's true, and we can avoid a colostomy [artificial means for elimination of body waste] for a patient.

HLN: And in advanced lung cancers you might help avoid hemorrhages and infections.

SL: Right. We can often relieve a cough, pain, coughing up blood, that sort of symptom, with radiation therapy.

HLN: Chemotherapy is usually considered much harder on the patient than radiation therapy.

SL: Chemotherapy in general has widespread effects which are usually more severe than radiation therapy. I think that is because you are dealing with a systemic method of treatment in chemotherapy as opposed to a local treatment with radiation.

HLN: Do you recommend a special diet for patients getting radiation therapy which may reach part of the gut?

SL: Our recommendation has always been to eat a diet which is low in residue, which means that we try to have a patient avoid fresh fruits, fresh vegetables, and any kind of roughage, like bran and other things which might irritate the bowel. Generally speaking, most patients can come through that treatment without any real serious or severe side effects.

HLN: Are they given any nutritional supplements?

SL: We recommend vitamins and we recommend frequent meals. I like for them to have malted milk, milk shakes, ice cream, and food of that nature.*

HLN: And do you have a particular emphasis on supplements?

SL: Not really, unless they're really losing weight. That has really not been a serious problem in most of the patients that we have treated.

---

* Needless to say, Dr. Levitt and I are in sharp disagreement on this point.

HLN: What do you have to offer a patient if his cancer has spread throughout his body?

SL: We can offer relief of symptoms, relief of pain.

HLN: How does radiation relieve pain, by shrinking the tumor?

SL: It does shrink the tumor, right; actually, it destroys cancer cells. A lot of bone pain, for instance, is caused by the tumor pressing against the periosteum [the tight connective tissue that surrounds all bones]. By shrinking the tumor we relieve the pressure and swelling and relieve the pain. Patients who have cancer spread to the spinal cord and have become partially paralyzed can achieve relief of that paralysis with irradiation. That is very important to a patient.

I think it's important to get this sort of data down. We can substantiate our opinions pretty well. There are too many emotional statements and misleading statements that only confuse and upset patients, and that's really unfortunate.

HLN: One point that you made that I think is very important: Patients should get a therapeutic radiologist on the team and have his opinion early in the game.

SL: I think that is extremely important.

HLN: How does one find a reliable radiological oncologist?

SL: People can check with their county medical society or local radiological society. The larger hospitals that are accredited by the JCAH [Joint Commission on Accreditation of Hospitals] and that have a tumor registry usually have a good team.

HLN: You think patients with cancer should see a therapeutic radiologist in consultation prior to surgery?

SL: I feel that's very important. Once the diagnosis has been made and before definitive treatment has been decided upon, it is essential for the patient to have a consultation with a therapeutic radiologist. He often has something valuable to add.

HLN: Is there anything else you want to tell the general public?

SL: The main thing is that cancer is not a hopeless

disease. Radiation therapy doesn't mean the end of the trail. About 50 percent of the cancer patients will be treated sometime during their illness with radiation therapy. And about half of those patients treated with radiation therapy will be treated mostly with success for cure. Many advances are being made: advances in radiation alone, advances in conjunction with chemotherapy or with surgery. (For example, as I mentioned, soft tissue carcinoma.) This has been a whole new area that's just opened up, with decreased morbidity and disability and excellent cure rate. Things are developing in cancer treatment which will help patients go on and live their lives in comfort with less disability than before.

IV

Diet, Vitamins, and Cancer

14

Robert Good: Research on the Relationship between Nutrition and Cancer

Sometimes when I request an interview with a doctor he will ask me to submit the questions two weeks in advance. I'm always a bit distrustful of that type of "authority." If he needs two weeks to look up the answers, he doesn't have the kind of information I want. I am always seeking firsthand experience. If it's not on the tip of their brains, then what they know isn't for me and my audience. Dr. Good didn't ask for a list of questions.

I knew a few things about Dr. Robert A. Good before I met him. He has spent many years doing fundamental work on the relationship between diet and cancer. He is one of the most respected men in the entire field of medicine and has been recognized by his colleagues by being appointed the Director of Research, Memorial Sloan-Kettering Cancer Center, and President and Director of Sloan-Kettering Institute for Cancer Research. You can't get much closer to the cancer section of Medical Heaven than that.

One of my teachers in grammar school used to tell us that a neat room and a neat desk meant a neat mind. During my visits with the important scientists I have interviewed for this book, I haven't seen a single neat room or one neat desk. My old teacher would be wrong if she concluded they didn't have neat minds, however.

Dr. Good's large, carpeted office in the modern skyscraper of the Center was stacked precariously high with slides and books and papers. We had to wade very carefully between the stacks to plug in my tape recorder.

There's usually a certain tension between doctors who are involved in teaching and research and those in private practice. The former tend to think they are the true medical gift to mankind and that practitioners are only rather obtuse money grabbers, while the latter often refer to those in academic circles as impractical and unable to make the grade in private practice.

I wondered how it would go between Dr. Good and me.

We were joined by Gabriel Fernandes, M.S., a visiting investigator who was working with Dr. Good.

Dr. Good slumped down in his chair (my grammar school teacher certainly wouldn't approve of that either!) and smiled at me. His eyes were hooded, but he didn't look sleepy. In spite of his relaxed ways, I had the feeling that I was in the presence of a Force.

Even though he was Gown and I was Town, we hit it off right away by following the sensible path of mutual respect. We both felt secure enough not to need to put the other down. What a pity it can't always be that way!

Anyway, here is the interview. I enjoyed it, and I think you will, too.

INTERVIEW WITH DR. ROBERT GOOD

R. GOOD: I think the most interesting thing we've learned about vitamin C comes from the work of Boxer and Bachner.

They studied the Chediak-Higashi anomaly. This is a disease associated with a high frequency of fatality from infection. If the children live long enough, they also develop malignancies. The basic problem in that

154

disease is that the phagocytes, the monocytes, and neutrophils behave as if they're drunk. They can't migrate toward or zero in on a foreign particle. Their chemotaxis* has been known to be defective for a number of years and to be associated with several changes in the white blood cells. They don't have a steering mechanism. They don't have the cytoskeleton, the cytoplasmic tubules haven't developed properly. All you've got to do is to expose those cells in a test tube to ascorbate and they form nice tubules and then become very effective in their phagocytic activity. So if you treat the patient with ascorbate, it corrects the abnormality. So here's this inborn error, associated with a high frequency of infection, a high fatality, and a high frequency of cancer, that may now be cured by just giving vitamin C.

H. L. NEWBOLD: So the work on vitamin C and cancer doesn't come as a big surprise to you.

RG: Well, I knew about Pauling's work long before the Boxer and Bachner work. But now the real sixty-four-dollar question is, will this treatment both prevent infection and the development of cancer? I bet it will.

HLN: What implications does this have for preventing and treating other types of cancer?

RG: I think that there may be cytostructural abnormalities associated with many forms of cancer. That's what some of the doctors here at Memorial Sloan-Kettering have been finding.

HLN: Then this may tie cancer in with ascorbic acid.

RG: Could be. It could give a rationale. I wouldn't want to say so at this point.

HLN: There's a possibility?

RG: The possibility exists. But let me finish what I was saying. The cytoskeletal structural correction is being associated with a correction of another marked abnormality in the patients with Chediak-Higashi di-

---

* Ability of white blood cells to travel to the site of injury upon chemical stimulation.

sease. The gigantism of the granules, for example. The cytoskeleton is very important for delivering in the proper way the granules to the outside of the cell.

HLN: What levels of ascorbic acid are you talking about?

RG: They're not huge, a little more than we ordinarily recommend, but they're not massive doses such as Pauling talks about. It's a very interesting association with a nutrient and possible susceptibility to cancer.

HLN: What do you think of Cameron and Pauling's work on vitamin C and cancer?

RG: I think it's not definitive. They've got a long way to go from these observations to real proof that vitamin C is effective in cancer treatment. So far they haven't done their work in a way that is convincing to me. I think it's an interesting preliminary observation. It's worth at least a proper double-blind controlled study.

HLN: But you can't get around the fact that 18 of the 100 treated patients were still alive at the end of five years and that all of the 1,000 untreated patients were dead at the end of that period.

RG: Yes, but I think that the study wasn't set up with proper controls.

HLN: Specifically what?

RG: An awful lot of patients with cancer can live five years. Eighteen out of 100 is not great for any of the kind of cancers that he's talking about.

HLN: But none out of 1,000?

RG: That may not be representative.

HLN: How do you mean?

RG: Eighteen percent five-year survivals is not an inordinate figure for many cancers without treatment.

HLN: But these were terminal cancers.

RG: That's a judgment. The really aberrant figure is the zero in 1,000. If you study cancer patients as we see them around here, it would be really strange to have none of 1,000 cases that we called advanced cancer surviving five years. So I think the figure that's more like the general experience is the 18 of 100.

HLN: Well, these were judged to be terminally ill.

RG: Well, you see so often with terminally ill cancer patients something happens and they go for a long time. It depends on the kind of cancer.

HLN: Why did none of the 1,000 controls go a long time, I wonder. More than five years?

RG: I don't know. But I still insist that that is an interesting preliminary observation. It is not definitive. Simultaneous randomly related controls are necessary. And it needs a properly controlled study; that is, there may be errors of acquisition to that study. There may be problems of acquisition, I don't know. But you have to have set it up so that the cases are randomly assigned and then see whether it works.

HLN: Well, still eighteen against zero would have to be highly selective.

RG: Yes, chance alone probably is not operating, but I don't know yet that it was their treatment that produced the effect.

HLN: Very unlikely that chance alone . . .

RG: Right, but I'm not sure chance alone was operating unless you set it up in a proper way. That's the only criticism. You've got to be very, very critical of these things.

HLN: What work are you doing here in regard to nutrition and cancer?

RG: We've got a big program on nutrition and cancer. We're of course very much interested in man and the associations between nutrition and cancer.

HLN: What do you think about Cameron's talk about resistance to cancer?

RG: I'm sure there is such a thing as resistance to cancer.

HLN: Do you think there is such a thing as natural resistance?

RG: Oh, sure. I think we don't yet know the basis of it, however.

HLN: Partly it's hereditary. But what about nutrition? Does nutrition have anything to do with resistance?

RG: I think nutrition has an awful lot to do with resistance.

HLN: In what way?

RG: Gabriel Fernandes and I have been studying this experimentally. We can take mice with the proper genetic determinants, the proper hormonal makeup, and a known virus determinant of breast cancer. We can reduce the occurrence of breast cancer from 70 to 80 percent in those mice to zero.

HLN: By doing what?

RG: Just cutting calories from the time of weaning.

HLN: And what calories do you cut—the fats or carbohydrates?

RG: It doesn't make any difference, so far as we can tell. But there needs to be a lot more study on that.

HLN: It's known that obese people get cancer more frequently than slender people.

RG: Certain kinds, anyway.

HLN: What kinds?

RG: Breast cancer, for example.

HLN: What about vitamins, minerals, and so forth? What do they have to do with resistance?

RG: I think a lot, but it hasn't yet been very well studied. Very careful studies have shown that if you restrict the intake of vitamin B_6 you very much interfere with cell-mediated immunological responses* that are virus dependent. That was work done by the Fishers a number of years ago.

HLN: And the same thing is true of vitamin C deficiency, isn't it?

RG: Vitamin C deficiency does have influences on immunologic functions, but there have not been what I consider definitive studies on that with modern technology.

HLN: There have been some studies with vitamin A, too, haven't there? What about them?

---

*The immunological system helps fight cancer. Certain vitamins and minerals help that system work more effectively. —H. L. N.

RG: Well I think they show associations that have to be investigated; however, I don't think either vitamin A or vitamin C has been definitely investigated. There is much exciting evidence that maybe vitamin A can prevent some cancers.

HLN: Do you consider them promising?

RG: Absolutely. We're doing a lot of work here with trace metals and their associations with malignancy and immunological function.

HLN: Could you tell me about that?

RG: About 1970, some fellows in Denmark discovered a lethal mutant in cattle (called the A46 mutant) which is associated with skin lesions, gastrointestinal malfunction, and very markedly increased susceptibility to infection and early death. This was associated with a severe deficiency of cell-mediated immunity and was corrected simply by giving zinc. Those cattle had inherited an inability to absorb zinc normally through the gastrointestinal tract. Without zinc they couldn't survive. They had a lethal disease. When Brummerstedt, Andresen, and Flagstad studied the basis of that disease, they found a profound deficiency in certain immunological functions. The thymus was very small and poorly developed. That was an interesting observation.

I think it was in 1973 that Moynahan discovered that the highly morbid and frequently lethal acrodermatitis enteropathica in humans could also be cured by giving relatively large amounts of zinc by mouth. That disease, an inborn error of metabolism transmitted as a recessive trait, causes central nervous system malfunction, skin lesions, gastrointestinal lesions, and profound deficiencies of immunological function in children. The children frequently died of infection before we knew enough to give them zinc.

Their disease is very, very similar to the A46 lethal mutant in cattle. Here's a rare, genetically determined immunodeficiency disease curable by just giving a simple element. If you take the element away, the kids get their awful disease back. It's really pretty dramatic. Children with that disease are difficult to live with. They look away, they're very fussy and irritable, they've even been called autistic. Within hours after giving zinc you've started to correct, then cure that central nervous system malfunction; within weeks you cure the gastrointestinal and skin lesions, and within several weeks their immunological functions return to normal.

We've now produced that disease in experimental animals, mice and rats, simply by taking the one element, zinc, out of the diet.

We've now studied this problem with modern immunological techniques. The natural killer cells that may be associated with defense against malignancy, the T-cell-mediated immunities that we can produce by immunizing with tumor cells, the ability to form antibodies to thymus-dependent antigens, all of that is deficient in the animals fed a diet deficient in zinc. The thymic hormone levels, which we can now measure in the circulation, fall to a very low level, and the lymphoid system looks like the lymphoid system of a thymectomized animal.

All of this syndrome and all of the abnormalities of the lymphoid system are immediately and promptly correctable just by giving the animals the single element zinc. The importance of this, of course, is that immunodeficiency very frequently occurs in patients with cancer. And already in many patients with cancer we find low levels of serum zinc.

HLN: I've done thousands of zinc levels on patients. Very frequently I find a low zinc level in patients. I use the hair-analysis method to measure zinc as well as other mineral levels in each new patient who consults me.

RG: I think that the hair analysis, the urinary excretion, the salivary excretion are confirmatory, but too difficult; I think you can get all the information you need just from measuring the serum zinc, if you use really good methods. You've got to be very careful of your stoppers and tubes.

HLN: I've used both hair and serum zinc tests and find the hair tests more stable. You can walk up a flight of stairs, for example, and change your serum zinc level.

RG: That's a fascinating thing, and its effects on the immunity functions are profound! I'm having a love affair with zinc. But I think that other scientists investigating immunity ought to have a love affair with other trace metals like selenium, magnesium, manganese, cobalt and copper.

We have studied immunodeficient patients. We follow and study patients with hypogammaglobulinemia and many different forms of immunodeficiency. Sometimes these patients will get T-cell immunodeficiency as well. Doctors at Emery, discovered that such patients who also had skin lesions, gastrointestinal disorders, and T-cell abnormalities had low levels of zinc. And you can correct all the symptoms and findings of the T-cell deficiency just by giving them zinc.

HLN: You have studied zinc levels on people with active malignancies?

RG: It's too early to know the whole story, but there's no question that many patients with malignancies and some with immunodeficiencies have low zinc levels.

HLN: One question arises in treating neoplasms nutritionally. Since the malignant tissue itself has high levels of certain vitamins and minerals—it apparently robs the body of them—is it wise to give these nutrients to the patient? Think of folic acid, for example.

RG: The answer isn't known yet. The question is being studied now in several controlled experiments. I think that basically giving nutriments to patients with malignancies will probably be helpful, because it facilitates the effective use of chemotherapy. It's going to have to be established for each and every disease.

HLN: If it is true that resistance enters into the picture of the patient fighting his malignancy, then it would be logical to give the nutrients, but logic doesn't always work out.

RG: That's right. It's a little treacherous.

HLN: But of course there are patients who can't wait until we have all the answers. One hundred years from now we'll know, but what are you going to do in the meantime?

RG: Medicine has a long history of treating before it understood things completely, and sometimes it works.

HLN: In the event that you or someone in your family had a malignancy, would you give them folic acid and other nutrients? If the cards were down, how would you play the game?

RG: I think that I would probably use the nutrients. I would do it recognizing that it might be wrong.

HLN: I'm in a position where I have to play my cards every day. I'm not in the position that you're in.

RG: You asked about our studies on nutrition. We're doing many studies on the influence of parenteral nutrition in this institution. Dr. Shils here is doing an analysis of the influence of hyperalimentation, seeing whether this improves chemotherapy by lowering the risk of toxicity. He's using controlled studies to see if it benefits the outcome of the cancer patient.

Fernandes has been working with me for a number of years on the influence of many different nutrients on immunity functions and on the development of cancer. I got seriously interested in the relationships of nutrition and immunity when I made a trip to Africa in 1969 and visited my former student Galal Aref, who was then an associate professor of pediatrics at Alexandria University. There I encountered his studies of Palestinian refugee children who were grossly deprived of nutrients, calories and protein, from the time of birth because their mothers were deficient and the milk supply failed very early. The children were fed pretty much on rice water with a little anise flavoring. Those kids developed kwashiorkor [severe protein deficiency] or marasmus [deficiency of both calories and protein] * by the time they were six to seven months of age. We found many of them to be hypo-gammaglobulinemic or even agammaglobulinemic and

---

* In practice they were, in both cases, also deficient in vitamins and minerals.

grossly immunologically deficient.* Seventy-five percent of them were dying from infection. When you fed them adequate amounts of food, it took them quite a while to fully recover their immunologic functions. These important findings were evident even from the studies done with crude techniques at that time.

HLN: How long did it take them to recover?

RG: At six months to a year they still had demonstrable abnormalities. After two years of treatment they had pretty much recovered normal immunological functions. This was very provocative to me and made me really think deeply about the whole issue of nutrition and its effect on immunity.

Then I went on to Lake Victoria in East Africa, where my wife and I were collecting lungfish for our phylogenetic research. While there I was able to study kwashiorkor in East Africa, and especially the pathological material from patients who died of infection while they had kwashiorkor. There the problem with children was very different. There's no real shortage of food in East Africa. The problem there is that kids are shoved out of the nest by the following child and they have to struggle on their own to establish themselves in their ecological niche. They get nutritional deficiencies because protein is not nearly as readily available as carbohydrate. The short of a long story is that they very frequently have profound cellular immunodeficiencies, T-dependent immunodeficiency as well as antibody deficiency syndromes. Studying their tissues from a pathological perspective was just like looking at the children with combined immunodeficiency that I had studied so extensively earlier when they had died of measles. We found much evidence of virus infections, but very little evidence of resistance to the virus, in terms of inflammation and lymphocytes and plasmacytes. The mortality rate of measles in some of those kwashiorkor children may be as high as

---

* Because of poor nutrition, their immunological systems couldn't fight off infections and cancer efficiently.

80 percent, which is huge. It's up about 50 percent in most studies.

After these two clinical experiences I tried to determine the very best way to analyze the influence of nutriments on immunity. I just couldn't see how it could be done by studying malnutrition in the field. There is always so much infection and infestation in these children. All those things can affect immunity, plus the dietary deficiency. Further, what is called protein deprivation or protein–calorie deprivation is never simple and may be extremely complex, with associated vitamin deficiencies, trace metal deficiencies, and iron deficiencies, among other things.

Consequently, I decided we would have to study the problem in the laboratory and not only in the field. Fernandes had gone to work with Yunis in Minnesota at that time. He was very much interested because he had been studying the influence of nutrition on reproduction in chickens. He decided that he was going to help us to get our mouse colony going. We were trying to work with certain strains of mice that have very interesting, spontaneously occurring disease. One strain of these mice shows many if not all of the manifestations of diseases of aging very early in life, that is, during the second half of the first year of life. These are the mice of the NZB and NZBXNZW strains.* This was pretty crude work to begin with, because the diets weren't very well defined. We found that if you use a high-fat diet, probably also a high total caloric intake, the animals developed early and had more evidence of autoimmune disease, died earlier, and had an early onset and progression of what we call diseases of aging. By contrast, those on the lower fat intake lived longer and had less autoimmunity vascular disease and cancer. So we set up studies to really dissect these issues using completely defined diets. The studies have been going on for nearly ten years now, and the

---

* Certain inbred strains of mice. There are many such strains, each with special characteristics. Some develop breast cancer easily, for instance, others alcoholism, and so on.

results are just fascinating. Most dramatic effects have been produced by total caloric restriction from the time of weaning.

HLN: That's interesting, but when you're dealing with a rat you're dealing with an animal that is quite different nutritionally from a human being. A rat's natural diet is grain and a man's natural diet is meat. Biologically they are two very different creatures.

RG: Yes, but let me pursue this, because I'm convinced that what we are learning can be brought to the general case. In humans you have the situation where so-called protein–calorie malnutrition is associated with much cell-mediated immunodeficiency. In the mouse, the rat and the guinea pig, and in a few monkeys that have been studied, the caloric or protein restriction is associated instead with increased evidence of cellular immunity. In protein–calorie malnutrition, until you get down to the extremely low levels that influence appetite, you enhance the cellular immunity rather than depress it.

HLN: By reducing the protein intake to a certain level.

RG: Yes.

HLN: I do medical nutrition. People come to see me with all sorts of disorders and I treat them without medication, with nutritional approaches. Almost all the people I see do better on a high-meat, high-fat diet. They feel better, their hypertension goes away, they lose weight, they become less depressed, they have more energy, their headaches disappear, their arthritis goes away. All sorts of interesting things happen.

I can control their cholesterol levels. I can put everyone's cholesterol wherever they want it with lecithin or niacin or ascorbic acid or various other nutrients. They can eat all the fat they want. It is not a problem. I wonder why it is the people feel so much better on high-fat. You've got to have either fat or carbohydrates, because you can't make the calories on protein. Why do people feel so much better on fat than they do on carbohydrates?

RG: Well, I think to some extent we are intoxicating ourselves with excessive carbohydrates. I don't know why. But mostly from just eating too much.

HLN: I see the people who can't make it on the general diet. They're sick. And I'm sure that if you plotted people's ability to live on diets heavy with carbohydrates such as wheat and sugar you would get a bell-shaped curve. There are many people who do fairly well on a wheat-and-sugar diet, but there are an awful lot of people who can't hack that diet at all. Apparently their biology is just not set up for it. And I don't know why. It would be interesting to see what happens to their immunological status when they change diets.

RG: Thus far we have taken only toddling steps with our experimental work. Ultimately we hope to develop a real ability to manipulate and control the immunity system with lessons learned from our dietary manipulation. We have shown that minerals and vitamins, calorie intake, protein intake, fat intake can have profound influences on immunity functions. The great potential is that we are now working in model systems that can be dissected in immunological, cellular, molecular and hormonal terms.

HLN: The easiest way for the average person to control caloric intake is to have a diet high in fat and high in protein.

RG: Right.

HLN: Banting discovered this in 1864. There's something abnormal about an animal that gets fat on what it's eating.

RG: Very interesting. These mice, these autoimmune susceptible strains that develop all these diseases of aging—vascular disease, even coronary disease, kidney disease, and malignancy in high frequency—these animals are obese strains. If you feed them enough they'll eat enough to get fat, just like humans. If you give them a high fat intake they'll get very fat. If you give them a total calorie intake that's too much they'll get just roly-poly.

HLN: And if you cut the carbohydrate and just give them fat and protein, what happens?

RG: Well, we've tried that to some extent. The thing that really counted was the total amount of food that they took in.

HLN: But would they get fat on just fat and protein?

RG: I can't really say that for sure without carbohydrates in there. We just haven't studied that yet.

HLN: Well, I get fat if I eat all the carbohydrate I want. I can gain twenty pounds in a month.

RG: A number of mouse strains aren't obese. Without force-feeding they won't eat excessively. On the other hand there are strains that are obese, that will eat excessively, like humans. With this strain that eats excessively, if you give them too much to eat you shorten their life span very significantly, and you accelerate the development of what we have called the diseases of aging. If you restrict their caloric intake from early life, you double their life span. You can make the longest-lived of them live as long as the average of the strains of longest lived mice.

With people too I think that certain cancers may be facilitated by eating too much food. Some cancers seem to be influenced by eating too much meat. I think that these are interesting epidemiological associations that are not yet understood.

HLN: One thing that fascinates me about meat will interest you, I think. I have many patients who are highly allergic to food. And for some people it's important how meat is cooked. For example, if a steak is fried and subjected to high temperature on the surface, some people will be allergic to it, whereas if they boil it they're not allergic to it at all. The interesting thing is that I think gas broiling picks up hydrocarbons in the meat. I'm reasonably sure this contributes to the cancer statistics.

RG: We also know there are highly mutagenic chemicals that are created by pyrolation of the amines.

HLN: Right.

RG: So far the great impulse to carcinogenic chemicals has been the evolution of the plants and fungi.

And the second greatest impulse has been the introduction 10,000 to 50,000 years ago of fire. And now we're in the chemical revolution and we're introducing many more carcinogens. But we don't yet know how important their influence is going to be on production of cancer. Thus far, only three to five percent of cancers can be blamed on such chemical contamination.

HLN: By fire you mean the browning effect on meat?

RG: Yes, if you just take amino acid like tryptophane and you pyrolate that amino acid, as Takashi Sugimura has shown, with an appropriate application of heat, with a flame, you get as powerful a mutant as aflatoxin, which is the powerful carcinogen produced by funguslike aspergillus.

HLN: Why is it, I wonder—there's always an explanation for why we have biological urges—that meat tastes so much better when it's singed, when the surface is brown? People much prefer broiled meat to boiled meat. Why is that?

RG: I don't know. From an evolutionary point of view it's relatively recent.

HLN: We've had fire for 300,000 years but it only became popular around 50,000 years ago, relatively popular. But why do we prefer cooked food? I know we prefer cooked beans because raw beans will make us sick, but I don't know why we prefer cooked meat. Man does all right on raw meat.

RG: Well, I think that it really is the taste of the burned fat that contributes so much to the good taste of broiled meat.

HLN: I think I know why mankind likes sweets.

RG: Why?

HLN: It's been estimated that some 65 million years ago our ancestors lost the ability to manufacture vitamin C. With the loss of that ability came a propensity for sweets, which meant fruit in those days, so they would be assured of getting enough ascorbic acid. I think food manufacturers today have perverted that drive and turned it over to candy to make money out of it. When we eat sweets, I think, we're all really trying to get ascorbic acid. Patients who had allergic reactions suddenly develop a great desire for carbohydrates. For example, if you are allergic to perfume and get exposed to it, you immediately want carbohydrates. Many chemical insults make us want carbohydrates. Here again I suspect it's our attempt to get more ascorbic acid. Most animals—goats, for example—manufacture a great deal more ascorbic acid when they are under stress. I suspect it's in part a desire for ascorbic acid that makes many people obese when they go for sugar as a reaction to various stresses, emotional or allergic.

RG: Have you given them ascorbic acid in a controlled way so you really know?

HLN: I have observed that fat people under stress who want to go for candy can often block the desire for sweets by taking 10,000 milligrams or 20,000 milligrams of powdered vitamin C in a full glass of water.

There's one question I want to ask. Ascorbic acid is a great detoxifier, as you well know. There is a report, for example, of a patient unconscious from carbon monoxide poisoning getting intravenous ascorbic acid and waking up before the needle was removed. The question is, when you give ascorbic acid with chemotherapy for malignancies, are you going to protect the malignant cells as well as the healthy cells from the chemotherapy?

RG: I don't know. I think that's an interesting question.

HLN: I don't know either.

RG: I think you just have to test each of these questions with properly designed experiments. To some degree and for some things you can test with human cells in a test tube. We've got four hundred human cancer lines growing in the test tube, thanks to Dr. Fogh's work in this institute. You can look at that question right in the test tube for different kinds of cancer.

HLN: A physician named Saccoman in San Diego has treated about 50 patients with various malignancies with vitamin C. He has treated many of them at the same time they were receiving chemotherapy. His

opinion is that vitamin C does not block the chemotherapy. Patients do better with the combination. There
are three men in Japan who give chemotherapy, then
wait twenty-five minutes and give ascorbic acid. But
nobody knows the final answer.

RG: Well, I think those questions can be answered
rather quickly in the laboratory.

HLN: What else should the general public know?

RG: The other point that is so interesting in our experimental work is that we have been able to come in
even after all these diseases have started to develop
and still very much delay their progression.

HLN: What diseases?

RG: I'm talking about this animal-model system that
we've been using where you see the diseases of aging,
the kidney disease associated with autoimmunity, and
the decline of the immunological functions that I mentioned earlier.

HLN: By restricting calories?

RG: Yes. I think that's a very powerful effect. I
think that indicates it isn't absolutely necessary to
come in with the dietary manipulation at the very beginning.

HLN: And there's only one way to restrict calorie
intake in people that I know of, and that's to give them
a high-fat, high-meat diet.

RG: That helped me reduce, but I don't know if it
helped my vessels and my immunity system until I
study that issue directly.

HLN: I know that will do it. That and ascorbic
acid.

RG: But I'm not sure that we can even do this job
by dietary manipulation. I'm just not sure that we'll be
able to deliver what we discover any better than we
can deliver the knowledge that smoking cigarettes
causes cancer. Some smart people quit smoking and
they'll lose the risk they otherwise might have, but I
doubt if we can help the population as a whole very
much. So what I'm wondering is whether or not it isn't
just as important, or even more important, to learn how
our dietary influence is working so we have something

that can be delivered relatively simply. Now, I don't think there's any question one can deliver zinc to the individuals who would die if they didn't have zinc. I don't think there's any question that we can deliver ascorbic acid to the individuals who would die if they didn't have ascorbic acid. What I'm really wondering is whether we're not going to have to define the kind of information about major general dietary influence in cellular and molecular terms so that we will have something that is more readily deliverable. For example, by diet we can inhibit the involution of the thymus gland. We know that. We also know that the diseases of aging occur concomitantly with the loss of an efficient immunity system. That usually is associated with involution of the T-cell system. Maybe we can correct that defect simply by hormonal therapy. That's an interesting possibility.

HLN: What do you mean, hormonal therapy?

RG: We're already at the point of defining the thymic hormones. We're already at the point of actually translating initial observations on thymic hormones into a full understanding of the amino acid sequence of the peptide hormone, defining the active site and synthesizing the active site. That's what Goldstein thinks he has already accomplished, and I for one am much impressed by this data. It could be something as simple as that, it could be as simple as ascorbic acid. I would really like to think that if we understand these things and can get enough evidence from several different directions, people will be sensible enough to use the information, but you know it's only options that can be provided by science; options are not always picked up.

HLN: No. I recently talked with Szent-Györgyi— he's eighty-six years old . . .

RG: Yes, I know. He's a marvelous man. He has been most creative.

HLN: He said after he discovered the chemical structure of ascorbic acid he more or less lost interest in it. He used to take 1 gram a day. Last year he got pneumonia and couldn't seem to throw it off. He said he began to think maybe old men needed more ascorbic acid than young men. Then he upped his level to 8 grams and his pneumonia cleared away.

RG: Interesting observation. I just think it's a very heady experience to be able to double the life span, even of an animal. It doesn't matter to a scientist whose life span he doubles. To be able to control, with one relatively simple dietary maneuver, all of the things that I associate with diseases of aging is impressive to me. Autoimmunity, development of increased susceptibility to infection, development of malignancy, the development of vascular diseases, and the development of amyloid protein in the circulation are strongly influenced by a single maneuver.

HLN: Wouldn't it be interesting if one of the reasons people are fat is they're really trying to get more ascorbic acid for stress purposes? Perhaps that ties in with what you're saying.

RG: Those are interesting ideas. The Pauling postulates have not been tested in an immunological framework at all, to my knowledge. Pauling came here some years ago and told us his story—how he got his association with Cameron. The resistance to Pauling is largely a matter of his style.

HLN: Yes, he has to rush out to be public.

RG: Well, I don't worry about that. I think it's fine for the public to be talked to. He talks to them very effectively, but he hasn't yet taken his wonderful idea through the conventions of a well-defined scientific experiment that meets the criticisms of the most critical scientists and statisticians. I think he should. I think he owes it to the public to do that. But if he doesn't, some scientists will. I am sure of that, especially if Pauling states the hypothesis.

HLN: I don't know why he doesn't.

RG: Pauling has been one of the greatest geniuses of our century. He sees scientific problems and their solutions clearly when most of us cannot see what he is talking about. Thus, when questions tumble through my mind there may be not questions in his mind. But the rest of us have to proceed more conservatively with established steps. We don't think we can jump to the top of the mountain. We think we have to walk up slowly a step at a time.

HLN: People say the same thing about me, on a much smaller scale, of course. I have accumulated an enormous amount of clinical experience sitting across the desk day after day, year after year, from people who are sick and using nutritional techniques to solve their illnesses. I know what works with my patients, but to prove it to somebody else with control studies would be a monumental task. To start with, my personality isn't pointed in that direction. I get my kicks by helping sick people get well, not by performing experiments.

RG: The thing that the clinician does so beautifully is to throw out the questions. The scientists need those questions so they can subject them to experimental analysis with the hardest possible science and the most critical analyses possible.

HLN: To prove or disprove.

RG: Certainly. I often like to work with rare forms of diseases simply because I think we can utilize the questions asked by these diseases to gain understanding either by further laboratory analysis or further clinical investigation.

HLN: I think inborn errors of metabolism are extremely common. I think I see them in my office every day.

RG: Everybody is an individual, right.

HLN: Roger Williams has stressed, of course, that different people have widely different biological requirements. Much of our profession is entirely innocent of this idea, for some reason.

RG: Doctors aren't taught that kind of thing as well as they should be. We need to teach the science of nutrition very thoroughly.

HLN: It's inconvenient to have this knowledge, because it forces you to think about each patient. It's so much easier to call patients neurotic and write a prescription for Valium. I have patients whose lives have been changed by a certain vitamin or mineral. Sometimes I ask them, to what lengths would you go for vitamin C? And they say: "I would do anything to get it." They would actually kill for it, because they can't live anywhere near a normal life without it. These patients are not uncommon. I have a history professor who takes 6 mcg. a day of B_{12}. He can't function on less.

RG: Is that right?

HLN: By injection.

RG: I think you know more than I do about what we're talking about now. I don't know any scientific reason why such huge doses are needed. I would not reject the postulate out of hand, but I am skeptical.

HLN: Well, your thing and my thing are really very close, except we approach it from different directions.

RG: Yes, but that's fine. People are different. And I see a few things that are buried where other scientists wouldn't see them.

HLN: In what way?

RG: That's the lovely thing about individuality. Everybody sees things in a framework that he can handle. I happen to see things a bit differently from Linus Pauling and from you. Working together, as part of the whole of science, we sometimes discover things that neither one of us would discover alone.

HLN: Do you find others here interested in your nutritional studies?

RG: I think so.

HLN: That's interesting, because so often doctors in our society are uptight about everything having to do with nutrition.

RG: I know, but I've not encountered that. I have talked at all manner of medical meetings and scientific symposiums and scientific meetings all over the world. I find people fascinated with the subject of nutrition and wanting to know what the next thing will be that we can establish by our scientific analyses.

Remember Cartier when he was on that expedition in Canada? His troops were dying of scurvy. The Indians taught them to boil pine needles and to use the tea to cure their scurvy. That wasn't a controlled study, but it was the first real evidence of the power of a natural product to prevent and reverse a very lethal disease.

HLN: I used to think the medical profession would get more interested in nutrition, but by and large they're very hostile towards it.

RG: But haven't doctors always been resistant to new ideas? Medicine is and should be quite conservative. I think the burden is on us to give the information to them in a form that they can really understand and accept because we make it so clear and convincing.

HLN: Just because I tell them so is no reason for them to take my word for it.

RG: That's right. I wouldn't want them to accept my word or any of my hunches. I would want them to challenge and criticize and force me to do the right experiments, or do the experiments themselves.

HLN: I've been on TV and radio with professors of nutrition. They seem to have no practical knowledge of nutrition whatsoever. I mean they haven't worked with patients using nutritional techniques to treat their illnesses. One of them even said people should eat more sugar—fantastic.

RG: Well, that doesn't work for me. I feel lousy if I eat much sugar.

HLN: Well, perhaps on this note of agreement we ought to call it quits for the day.

RG: It was nice talking to you.

HLN: I'm very grateful for your time.

BIBLIOGRAPHY

Fernandes, G., P. Friend, E. J. Yunis, and R. A. Good, *Proceedings of the National Academy of Sciences U.S.A.*, vol. 75, no. 3, pp. 1500–1504, March 1978.

Fernandes, Gabriel, Robert A. Good, and Edmond J. Yunis, Chapter 9 in T. Makinodan and E. Yunis, eds., *Immunology and Aging*. New York: Plenum Medical Book Co., 1977.

Fernandes, G. E. J. Yunis, and R. A. Good. *Nature,* vol. 263, no. 5577 pp. 504–507, October 7, 1976.

Willis-Carr, J. I., and R. L. St. Pierre, *Journal of Immunology,* vol. 120, pp. 1153–59, 1978.

15

A Modern-Day Horror Story

We tend to think of malnutrition as something that happens only to poor people in central Mali or in the slums of Calcutta.

Not so. Starvation often shows its ugly face even in the fashionable sections of New York. The man I am about to tell you about was affluent. The reason he suffered from malnutrition was not because he lacked money to buy good food.

He was malnourished because his very expensive physicians were not taught about nutrition in medical school. His is, I am sad to say, a very common case, especially among patients suffering from cancer.

This is not a composite picture of a hypothetical patient but a true story about the treatment one man had for cancer. He was a man with a national reputation whose name many of you would recognize. Before his last illness he had been a nonsmoker, a nondrinker, a happy person who worked hard and enjoyed life, a man with intelligence and wit who was a pleasure to visit. I knew him only toward the end of his life, and not as his doctor, but I have assembled the facts about his illness.

He had seven doctors. Count them: a hematologist, a hypnotist, an internist, an oncologist, a psychiatrist, a radiologist, and a urologist. His final illness lasted from 1971 to 1978 and, in addition to what his health insurance paid, cost approximately $278,000. He was treated in New York at Columbus Hospital, Doctors Hospital, and Columbia-Presbyterian Hospital. A private hospital room cost $420.00 a day. Most of his doctors were on the teaching staff at Columbia University Medical School.

Let me make one thing clear: There was no question of negligence involved on the part of the doctors or the hospitals. This patient received the best standard medical care available. He was treated "by the book."

I simply want to show you readers how inadequate the best cancer treatment can be when the nutrition of the patient is ignored. Believe me, nutrition is ignored by most physicians.

As we go along, I will point out step by step how proper nutrition could have contributed to the patient's well-being.

1971

The patient had a transurethral operation on the prostate gland because of difficulty in urination. The microscopic sections showed the gland was cancerous.

The first nutritional error occurred when the surgeon came to the patient's room to tell him that he had cancer. The doctor pulled a cigarette out of his pocket and handed it to the patient. "You'll need this," he said.

Mind you, the patient was a nonsmoker until this point. He was introduced to the smoking habit by his doctor!

The patient soon became a four-pack-a-day cigarette smoker. Why, you might ask, is that so bad? After all, he already had cancer.

Here's why. Each cigarette smoked uses up about 25 milligrams of the body's supply of vitamin C. This means that this patient would need 2 grams of vitamin C daily just to stay even with the amount of vitamin C destroyed by his cigarettes.

The patient took no vitamin C during his entire illness, and generally ate foods that were devoid of the vitamin. There is every reason to think he was severely deficient in vitamin C all during his illness. Here is the clinical evidence he exhibited for a vitamin C deficiency.

1. The patient was severely depressed—suicidally depressed—during most of his illness. You might say that a man with cancer has a reason to be depressed. True, but when depressions are severe, as in this case, they are, in my experience, not generally due to psychological causes. Interestingly, this man's depression was not helped one iota by psychotherapy or antidepressant drugs. If the depression were psychological in origin, you would think one of these two treatments would have been helpful. You would expect the average patient to become more philosophical about his illness as time passed. He only grew more depressed.

I think his depression was caused in large part from a lack of vitamins and minerals, especially a lack of vitamin C. We know that in the eighteenth century, before we learned that lime juice both prevented and cured scurvy, sailors developed severe depression before they developed the full-blown picture of scurvy.

In my practice I rather frequently see depressed patients whose blood tests reveal a deficiency in vitamin C. When they are given vitamin C in adequate amounts, these patients usually lose their depression.

I think there is an excellent chance this patient's depression would have lifted if he had been given vitamins and minerals in adequate amounts.

His psychiatrist maintained the depression was "all in his head."

I think his psychiatrist was wrong.

At any rate, working on the assumption that it was "all in his head" did not enable the psychiatrist to cure or even alleviate the feeling of great hopelessness that engulfed the patient.

2. In the latter years of this patient's illness, he had repeated bladder hemorrhages.

It is well known that cancer victims do not usually die of cancer, but rather die of infection, hemorrhage, or starvation. Excessive bleeding is one of the cardinal signs of a vitamin C deficiency. Apparently this did not occur to the patient's doctors. None of them suggested that he stop smoking or start taking massive amounts of vitamin C.

3. Weakness is an important sign of vitamin C deficiency. This patient was extraordinarily weak during the last years of his illness. Radiation therapy, chemotherapy, poor diet, and cancer itself contributed to this weakness. But I would bet roller skates to a Rolls-Royce that his strength would have been greatly increased had he been given massive amounts of vitamin C along with all the other needed vitamins and minerals.

Incidentally, it has been well documented that stresses such as cancer, surgery, radiation, and chemotherapy also tend to deplete the body of vitamin C.

4. Loss of appetite was later suffered by this patient. This is also one of the symptoms of extreme vitamin C deficiency. Admittedly, there were other contributors to this problem, but a low vitamin C level could certainly have been a major contributor.

5. Marked swelling of the ankles occurred. Lack of capillary competency is a prime sign of vitamin C deficiency.

The patient was given the standard treatment for cancer of the prostate: female sex hormones. This is an effective way to slow down the growth of prostatic cancer in 80 percent of the cases. Often it gives the patient several years relatively free of cancer symptoms.

1972

Except for a gradually increasing depression, this was not a bad year for the patient. He began courting a former friend in December 1972.

1973

The patient married early in this year. Frequently, male patients are rendered impotent when given female sex hormones, but this was definitely not true in this case.

However, about three months after his marriage the patient gradually developed a much deeper depression.

It is of interest to note here that many authorities, including Dr. Good of Sloan-Kettering Memorial Cancer Center (see Chapter 14), have observed that zinc levels are low in cancer patients, and many think that zinc might well be important in the prevention and treatment of cancer. Carl Pfeiffer has repeatedly pointed out the importance of adequate zinc levels for the prevention and treatment of emotional symptoms.[1]

Since zinc is present in seminal fluid in large amounts, ejaculations tend to deplete the body of this mineral.

When the patient was first married he was quite active sexually. Seminal fluid is rich in zinc, so each ejaculation depletes the body of that mineral. He had a very poor diet that was low in zinc. It is quite reasonable to conclude that his body zinc levels were low before marriage and became much lower after marriage, hence contributing to both the spread of cancer and his depression. Certainly, a nutritionally astute physician would have measured the patient's zinc levels and administered a supplement of zinc if it was indicated.

Stress—any stress, whether it be a severe burn, a broken leg, anxiety, or even sex—lowers the body's levels of zinc and vitamin C. Certainly the first months of marriage are a period of stress. The whole situation would tend to lower the patient's zinc and vitamin C levels even more.

It is interesting to note that just before a biological system fails, it often has a great urge toward reproduction. This must be nature's way of trying to preserve the species even though the individual is about to die. Whether the perception of imminent death is mental or physical, it spurs sexual activity. We all know that soldiers about to be sent overseas or into battle experience a great drive toward sexual activity. Before patients have a nervous breakdown and sink into a state of near nothingness, they frequently go through a period of sexual frenzy.

One theory explaining the high birthrate in under-developed countries is that poor nutrition pushes these people toward reproduction before they die or become old before their time and incapable of sex.

We see this struggle to reproduce before death even in the plant kingdom. For example, when grasses are poorly nourished and are about to die, they go to seed. Again nature is trying to preserve the species, even though reproduction may deplete the individual and hasten its demise.

At any rate, about three months after his marriage the patient's condition rapidly deteriorated. He became tired and sank much deeper into his depression.

From this point on until he died, in 1978, the patient's life was a trail of utter misery. I have every reason to believe that with proper nutritional therapy these could have been good years. It is also quite possible that his life could have been considerably prolonged with proper nutritional help.

So far as I have been able to learn, his physicians did no vitamin and mineral studies on this patient (except perhaps for blood measurements of potassium and sodium). We can assume he was severely deficient in both vitamins and minerals. Not only was he smoking a vitamin-C-depleting four packs of cigarettes a day, but his diet consisted of carbohydrate foods largely deficient in vitamins and minerals.

He drank one to one and a half quarts of sugar-laden root beer daily while living mostly off salted popcorn, salted peanuts, salted potato chips, salted french fries, and salted pork products. He had a great craving for salt. This may well have been due to the beginning of failure of his adrenal cortical glands. It is well known that under stress the body tends to pour out more hormone from this gland. Perhaps his adrenal cortical glands were becoming exhausted at this point. People with failure of these glands feel somewhat better if they have a high salt intake. Interestingly enough, the adrenal cortical glands contain the body's highest concentration of vitamin C. Both vitamin C and pantothenic acid (one of the B vitamins) are especially important for the glands' proper functioning. Vitamin C is especially important in helping the body's defense against certain cancers, including cancer of the prostate.

Because of his diet, the patient was surely also deficient in vitamin B_{12}, folic acid, vitamin A, vitamin E, and the entire B complex. A deficiency of vitamin B_{12}, folic acid, and the B complex can also contribute to depression and tiredness.

The patient was also fond of lollipops and ate a great many. Here again he was turning to sugar, calories empty of protein, vitamins, and minerals. His desire for sweets such as sugared root beer and lollipops illustrates another interesting point about vitamin C. Humans are one of the very few mammals unable to make their own vitamin C. A 150-pound goat, for example, makes about 13 grams a day, and under stress its body may make three or four times this amount. This characteristic of animals making more vitamin C when under stress, coupled with clinical observations, leads us to believe that we humans also need more vitamin C when we are under stress, such as increased sexual activity, surgery, chemotherapy, radiation therapy, vitamin-mineral deficiency, and so on.

Irwin Stone estimates that our distant ancestors lost their ability to manufacture their own vitamin C about 65 million years ago, when they lived in the African forests, where their diet was largely fruit. Since their food was giving them an adequate amount of vitamin C, nature saw no need to use chemical machinery to produce this vitamin. Since then, we humans have been forced to depend upon diet for the daily supply of vitamin C.

At the same time we lost our ability to manufacture vitamin C, we had implanted in us a desire for sweets. In those days there were no candy bars or ice-cream parlors. Sweets meant fruit, which meant vitamin C. The desire for sweets, in other words, insured that we would get a constant supply of the much-needed vitamin C.

If animals under stress respond by manufacturing three or four times as much vitamin C as in nonstressful times, how do humans—who cannot manufacture vitamin C at all—get more vitamin C when under stress?

We all know that under stress we humans tend to want to eat sweets. We feel depressed and want more sweets. We have a hard day at the office and want pie and ice cream after dinner. We get an allergic reaction and want sweets.

Our desire for added sweets when we are under stress is nature's way of trying to see that we get extra amounts of vitamin C during those times.

But civilization has twisted the whole thing around. Now, instead of eating fruit to get the extra amount of vitamin C our bodies want, we eat something made with sugar, which gives us no vitamin C.

I strongly suspect that the patient's urgent desire for sweets was due to his body's trying to get more vitamin C. He was starving for it. Nature urged him to eat sweets, but to nature sweets means fruits and hence vitamin C. Instead, he ate sugar sweets and only depleted his body all the more of vitamins and minerals.

1974

Because of the spread of cancer, the patient was started on deep radiation and chemotherapy. This knocked him for a loop and robbed him of what little quality of life he had left. He became very nauseated, lost much weight, and was so weak he could hardly move about.

After the start of radiation and chemotherapy the patient awakened every morning for the next four years crying, hysterical, in total panic. He became, and remained for the rest of his life, suicidally depressed.

Until his death, he went into the hospital periodically for four-day chemotherapy treatments.

1976

The horrors continued. Because of increased pain, he was given more radiation therapy. Eventually the patient developed a chronic weeping open sore at the base of his spine due to radiation burn.

(Let me add here that every doctor I have talked with who has used massive amounts of vitamin C in the treatment of cancer has stressed how valuable it is for relieving the pain associated with cancer.)

During this year the surgeon removed the patient's testicles in an attempt to hold back the spread of cancer. The patient also had two operations on his bladder. I've already mentioned that the stress of surgery depletes the body of vitamin C and zinc.

1977

Because of the patient's constant nausea, he lost weight until he looked like an escapee from Buchenwald. Every bone in his body seemed to be trying to punch through his skin. Even his height shrank, so that by the end he had gone from 6 feet 5 inches to under 5 feet 10 inches.

At this point the patient received the only nutritional advice given during his seven-year illness—his internist suggested that he drink a chocolate-flavored nutrient!

It only made him more nauseated.

He started vomiting regularly. He began having massive hemorrhages from the bladder.

Of course, the hemorrhages only depleted his vitamin C, zinc, iron, and other vitamins and minerals all the more.

His lower legs swelled very badly (probably due in part to a lack of vitamin C), and he developed chronic cracks and sores on the bottoms of his feet. He was unable to wear shoes and could get about only in a wheel-chair.

Because of his great pain he was put on a "Bronford cocktail," a painkiller originated in England, consisting of a mixture of cocaine and morphine.

This really put him out of his head. Most of the time he was completely confused. He thought his wife was his mother. The painkiller never gave him any lift. It only made him out of touch, and, worse, greatly suppressed his appetite, causing him to waste away even more.

The morphine in the cocktail also increased his already dreadful constipation. To have a bowel movement he had to take two bottles of magnesium citrate plus two bottles of Fleet's enema mixture.

1978

The torturous downhill road continued until the patient's merciful death in the spring. I have been told that his death was not a natural one, that he was "helped along."

In Conclusion

That, my friends, is one man's story of cancer. He was given 278,000 dollars' worth (in addition to what the insurance paid) of the best medical care from seven of the country's better doctors.

But he was given no nutritional therapy whatsoever.

One of his doctors had the gall to claim on a talk show that he was especially interested in the nutritional status of patients and tested them for vitamin levels when indicated.

I wonder why he did not think such tests were indicated with this patient.

I strongly feel that proper nutritional therapy, such as I advocate in this book, would have completely altered the course of this man's illness. One of the characteristics of vitamin C therapy is that the patient feels good, suffers little pain, and often leads a normal life up until several weeks before death.

And, of course, it is possible death would have been postponed had this patient received adequate nutritional help. You will remember that Cameron and Pauling reported that 90 percent of their vitamin-C-treated patients lived three times as long as the untreated patients and 10 percent of them lived twenty times as long.

But once more let me emphasize, the *quality* of the patients' lives was greatly increased by the use of vitamin C.

A life of misery is of no value to anyone.

One of the sad things about this patient is that his name will go down in the book of statistics as a success for chemotherapy and radiation therapy because he lived seven years after a diagnosis of cancer was first made. Nonsense! For all practical purposes he was dead during those seven years, a wasted shell of a man who was a despair to himself and all those around him.

And to think that in all probability it could have been otherwise! With proper nutritional therapy, including massive amounts of vitamin C, he probably could have had seven good years—maybe more.

16

The Importance of Nutrition in Cancer Treatment

The last time I was in a dean's office was in 1942, when as an anxious freshman medical student, I stood in front of the giant desk belonging to the master of my fate and heard him tell me I'd better spend a bit more time studying anatomy. He was right. I didn't like the anatomy professor and I didn't like the subject and I didn't spend as much time on it as I should. But if I was going to become a doctor I now jolly well knew I'd better settle down and master the subject.

This time when I visited the dean's office I was not going to speak to the master of my fate, and so was considerably more at ease. But Dr. Theodore Cooper is the kind of man who could put even a first-year medical student at ease. His vibes are firm but relaxed.

Years ago I had a picture in my mind of a successful big-city doctor: He would be thin and tense as he rushed about his daily work. During the day he would live on Dexedrine and coffee, and he would take a sleeping pill to knock himself out for a few hours at 1:00 A.M. Now that I am a fairly successful big-city doctor myself and have had many opportunities to observe others, I must say that, leaving out one or two rare exceptions, I have not found anyone to match my boyhood fantasy. Indeed, most of the men who get to the top in their fields are sober, easygoing leaders who are not threatening toward their fellow man. And they usually give a baker's dozen.

Ted Cooper is a big-city doctor who immediately puts you at ease and treats you as if he has all the time in the world to devote to your interests. When he talks you realize at once that he has broad interests in the medical world and is in good command of the over-all picture.

As Dean of the Cornell University Medical College, he is one of the country's important medical educators. I would feel more comfortable about the future of the profession if he were in charge of all the medical schools.

I still think of Cornell's medical school buildings as gleamingly new, but, like Rockefeller Center, they are maturing. The dean's office, with its dark mahogany furniture and generation-and-a-half-old gray carpeting, shows that the place has begun to put some years behind it. Don't misunderstand me—I like it, and find it more comfortable now that time's mellowing hand has touched it.

Interview with Dr. Theodore Cooper

H. L. Newbold: I understand that you're interested in Vitamin C.

T. Cooper: I have no special research experience with vitamin C, but I became interested in it from a public health standpoint because of discussions with Dr. Pauling. We have had discussions about the use of vitamin C to treat viral diseases, including the common cold, and the role of vitamin C in cholesterol metabolism. When we were designing programs with the National Heart Institute several years ago, the issue of vitamin C as an important nutrient kept coming up.

I was also informed about the use of vitamin C to treat terminally ill cancer patients by Dr. Pauling himself. He visited me and we discussed some of the studies he was doing in Scotland. So repeatedly I've had the issue of vitamin C brought to my attention in different ways.

HLN: This goes back to when?

TC: To about ten years ago.

HLN: This was before you were in governmental circles?

TC: No, I was in governmental circles. I was the director of the National Heart Institute when I first became aware of its broader uses. Of course, before that I knew about vitamin C in the general medical sense, as any physician would know about its historical relations with scurvy, but I didn't really think about it in its relationship to modern public health challenges until I did get into a governmental role in 1968.

HLN: Why has nothing come of it with the American Heart Association? Why have they not advocated vitamin C for lowering cholesterol levels, for example?

TC: I think there continue to be some studies involving it, but the information about cholesterol metabolism has grown rapidly in the last ten years. When you're dealing with large numbers of people who are not homogeneous you get into problems of evaluating clinical studies. I think there just hasn't been a definite conclusion yet about what might be the best way to lower cholesterol levels. Even cholesterol-lowering drugs that were designed and tested by the government have never really given a satisfactory answer. No study has demonstrated as yet that cholesterol-lowering drugs prevent or help cure coronary heart disease. So I think the whole field of pharmacologic or nutriental cholesterol-lowering techniques remains unclear, except in varied selected cases.

HLN: They have taken a stand for the Prudent Diet.

TC: It's difficult for me to see any objections to having people avoid obesity, which is the crux of the Prudent Diet.

HLN: Except that it doesn't work to control weight.

TC: Well, it works in some people. I've seen a few myself. Certainly, lowering weight will often revert high cholesterol levels back to normal.

HLN: Yes, but we all know that the best way to lose weight is to eat a high-protein diet.

TC: Yes.

HLN: Or even a high-fat diet.

TC: Well, you can lower weight different ways. A lowering of the total caloric intake does usually involve a relative increase in protein and decrease in fat and sugar in the diet. I'm speaking of refined sugars.

HLN: I have the feeling that governmental circles, the FDA and so forth, are generally hostile towards vitamin therapy. Is that correct?

TC: I don't think they're hostile. I was interested in the controversy about vitamin therapy. Some of the senators and the agency were concerned about claims that were excessive relative to the data available. They were worried about the advocation of megavitamin therapy in the absence of any data on possible harmful effects. I wouldn't consider that in the range of "hostile."

I got caught up in that controversy myself. A popular publication said that I took vitamin C. They asked why a senior government health official didn't practice what the agency preached. My response was that the agency's responsibilities were not my personal responsibilities. As a person, I had to make up my own mind about how to conduct my life. I don't think the government should prescribe for me personally. The government's basic role is protection. If the government offers what evidence it has, then I think that is appropriate.

HLN: In my view, one of the problems government has with the whole problem of vitamin therapy is that it refers to professors for information. I was recently on a TV program, for example, with a well-known professor of nutrition from Harvard. He has no real practical information about the treatment of medical disorders with diets and vitamins. He spent most of his life doing research in laboratories.

On the contrary, I make a living by sitting across a desk day after day, year after year, with people who come to me with high blood pressure or high cholesterol levels, one thing and another. I treat them nutritionally. The academic people haven't been in the bullpen, so to speak. The government gets much information from the people who really don't have good practical information to give, if you understand what I mean.

TC: Oh, I think what you say makes sense. I think with the government or with any group, there is a great tendency to go towards academia. The people who invite the opinions or establish advisory committees cannot tell by reading a curriculum vitae or a title whether these expert witnesses ever treat patients or not, much less how many patients or what kind.

HLN: These so-called experts often pretend to have knowledge which they in fact don't really have.

TC: Well, I think that they're not asked the specific questions that you raise. In certain clinical areas well-known figures are consulted who do see a lot of sick people and they do know of which they speak. So there is a mixture of information, but the point that you make is well taken. I think that a policy maker should seek the input from a practitioner himself.

HLN: Those of us in private practice see medical problems from a different viewpoint than the professor. What you learn from doing research on a rat may or may not be applicable to humans.

You take vitamin C yourself, you say. How much do you take?

TC: I don't take it as a fanatic. When I have my breakfast I take 500 milligrams.

HLN: Why?

TC: I was in surgical training for a while and I was interested in the effect of vitamin C on wound healing and blood clotting. We used it empirically, on the basis of some experimental evidence that indicated it would be helpful in certain clinical situations in the post-operative period. And, seeing it used pretty often, I became familiar with it.

HLN: Why do you take 500 milligrams when the Recommended Daily Allowance is now something like 60 milligrams?

TC: Well, because I have tablets in that size.

HLN: But you could have bought tablets in smaller sizes.

TC: I just felt that if I was going to take a supplement I would take one that I could handle. I tried a gram a day and got a little gastric irritation.

HLN: Where do you get your tablets?

TC: At a drugstore.

HLN: I worry about people who take the tablets. The tablets cause a lot of trouble. There is a research project at the Mayo Clinic on vitamin C and cancer. I'll bet the tablets are being used and there will be a lot of gastric irritation and diarrhea reported. If you go to your corner drugstore and get a handful of ascorbic acid tablets and take them in quantity, you're going to have diarrhea and gastric irritation. We find that most people tolerate the fine ascorbic acid powder best, because it has no binders. Apparently the binders in tablets cause a lot of trouble. This is a common problem. It is also a common problem that the government* falls over its feet because it doesn't seek advice from people who have had practical clinical experience.

TC: I think the point that you make about clinical input is well taken.

HLN: We find that some people tolerate the sodium ascorbate or the calcium ascorbate best. A few people tolerate the long-acting type best.

Are you worried about the toxicity of vitamin C?

TC: Well, I worry about toxicity with anything at certain levels. I don't know that much about it, the top end. I know from talking with Dr. Pauling that I'm not taking a large dose at all. I worry about the upset-stomach effect because I've experienced it, as I just mentioned. It's hard for me to believe that some level of vitamin C wouldn't be harmful, but I don't have any evidence against it. Just as a usual caution I would feel that there should be some sort of limit.

---

* The federal government is sponsoring the Mayo Clinic test.

HLN: There is a limit and people do get upset. They get the same toxic symptoms when they eat too many apples and oranges: bellyache, gas, and diarrhea. It's self-limiting. People have tried to commit suicide on vitamin C, but no one has ever succeeded.

TC: Well, it's probably a relatively innocuous substance.

HLN: Does your family take vitamin C?

TC: My family doesn't take anything, unless I put it out for them. If I make the effort in the morning to put out some vitamin C they'll take it. When one of them has a cold or looks a little under the weather, I urge them to take it. But my family's getting grown up now. They pretty much think for themselves.

HLN: Do you feel that the 500 milligrams a day has made any difference in your life?

TC: I don't know that I can prove anything, but I think I've had only two or three real colds in the past couple of years. I travel a lot and have long schedules. I certainly believe that the vitamin C isn't doing me any harm. On those days when I feel I'm going to be under greater stress I might take a gram. I have in the past. I haven't done any controlled studies, but I think it's been useful to me.

HLN: I'll have to send you some powder to try the next time you get a cold.

TC: That's when I get into difficulty. I start getting a cold, then try to take more ascorbic acid and end up with gas.

HLN: That is a common problem with the drugstore type of vitamin C tablet.

You talked to Pauling about cancer treatment with vitamin C. Do you have any opinions about that?

TC: He did not show me any real clinical data, though his observations certainly were interesting. Even if the results were fortuitous, they should be investigated further. I would be terribly surprised if in the management of cancer or any other serious chronic debilitating illness, good nutrition, including vitamin C, were not helpful. I am delighted to see a little more awareness of the importance of nutrition that's stemming from the discussions in Congress a couple of weeks ago. I believe that good nutritional adjutant therapy is important. I think we have not paid enough attention to the nutritional side of treating diseases.

HLN: Why has the medical profession ignored nutrition?

TC: It's been preoccupied with specific treatments for diseases.

HLN: Well, that is one way of ignoring nutrition.

TC: Yes, in a sense.

HLN: Neglected, perhaps we should say.

TC: Yes, I think nutritional therapy has been neglected because of the medical profession's great preoccupation with specific drug interventions. Doctors want to find the specific cause of a disease and treat that.

Another reason medicine has neglected nutrition is that it has never been presented to the young people in the profession as an intellectually exciting area for accomplishment.

Third, not enough doctors understand nutrition. It's hard to teach what you don't know. I think there's only an awakening awareness of the importance of nutrition in the education of American medical students, or any medical students. If you ask a medical student or a young house officer about diabetes or glycogen-storage disease he'll tell you a lot. But you ask them about nutrition as opposed to a specific metabolic disease, they'll say, "Oh, yes, we know about vitamins and the required daily allowances." They go through those things in a few lectures on chemistry, I suspect. They have no appreciation that nutrition has an intellectual base for solving problems of illness. Nutrition is looked upon as one of those background things. Everyone's got to eat. We know you have to have nutrition and there is such a thing as starvation and anorexia nervosa and all that, but nutrition as such has never really had the standing of other specialties in medical schools.

HLN: Are you doing anything to correct that situation?

TC: We have some fine resources that we are trying to bring to bear on the subject. Our parent university has an excellent school of agriculture and human ecology in the nutritional division. I have a high regard for them, and participated in their institute this summer. We have a group that is meeting between the two campuses to try to make more than just a paper agreement. We're going to enhance our resources here at the medical center. We will try to introduce people into our hospitals from their clinical nutrition programs, get them in a setting where they can work with the young doctors rather than stand on the sidelines. We have a department of public health and preventive medicine and have them involved in these discussions.

One of the problems is that the medical curriculum is very full these days. Everybody wants more of the medical students' curriculum time. The students, on the other hand, want more electives. We find ourselves with shortened hours and increasing demands and changing awareness. It is difficult to develop a fluid, dynamic curriculum that allows us to give the students more exposure to courses in nutrition. There's no question but that the administration and the leaders of this institution are beginning to think that more instruction in nutrition is important. It will be included more in the system, but it won't be instantaneous.

HLN: I've been always surprised at the reluctance of the medical profession to take the subject of nutrition seriously. Nutrition seems fundamental to me. We're always dealing with living tissue. Since living tissue must have nutrition, nutrition seems like the logical place to start. Patients come to me with anginal heart pain, high blood pressure, arthritis, emotional problems, and a host of other disorders. These things can all be handled nutritionally very satisfactorily, often with better results than by the drug route. There are many things you can do nutritionally that you can't do with drugs. The doctors treating with drugs pretend to be more sophisticated than they really are. When we are able to create human life in a test tube and sustain it, I will be impressed at how sophisticated we are biochemically. Until then, I am really not too impressed with our knowledge of biochemistry.

TC: But nutritional therapy and drug therapy need not be mutually exclusive.

HLN: No, they need not be, but unfortunately many times they are.

TC: Too often they're looked upon as alternatives rather than helpful things to be considered together. If we exclude the obvious—that a good nutritional base is critical in the management of any condition—then I think we make an error. We shouldn't exclude nutrition. I think that doctors either are taught or come to believe that a great deal of the things about megavitamin theory, special kinds of diets, and all this sort of thing smacks of quackery. They don't want to be smeared with something that might be quackery.

HLN: Well, there are some quacks in the field of nutrition.

TC: Yes, there are some quacks. When a patient comes in and all he gets is a shot of vitamin B_{12}, that doesn't help anybody's confidence that there is something valuable in nutritional therapy.

HLN: Well, not everybody needs a shot of vitamin B_{12}, but I take serum B_{12} levels on all of my new patients. I've had patients who have gone through Memorial Hospital in the University of North Carolina, who have gone through Yale New Haven Hospital, who have gone through the Columbia Hospital complex with symptoms stemming from a vitamin B_{12} deficiency, and all of those hospitals missed the diagnosis because they failed to test for a vitamin B_{12} deficiency.

TC: Well, I think vitamin B_{12} is a great agent and doesn't need to be apologized for, but if a nice lady comes in with a backache and the first thing she gets is an injection of B_{12} . . .

HLN: Well, that's not the way to do it.

TC: That's not the way to do it. It reduces credence. If you send a young medical student out to work with a doctor like that, he comes away without a proper understanding of nutrition.

HLN: I had something interesting happen to me the other day. A professor in the department of allergy at Mount Sinai happened to read one of my books. On his own he telephoned to say how much he had enjoyed the book, how correct it was, and so forth. I thanked him and said they were coming out with a paperback edition of it and asked if he would like to write an introduction for it.

He said he couldn't do that because his colleagues wouldn't understand and they might not refer any more patients to him.

TC: Well, he's giving it to you honestly. A physician's income is often determined by referrals, and if other doctors get the notion that he does peculiar things . . . well, he'll lose referrals—except perhaps in this town. There are doctors here who have very peculiar practices. They inject urine and do a variety of other things that are out-and-out quackery.

HLN: I don't particularly advocate auto-urine injections, but I have a collection of about forty medical papers from around the world advocating it. Apparently it's effective in treating some allergies.

TC: I don't doubt that there's something in urine that could be active in a variety of things, but it's hard to have young physicians accept something like that.

HLN: Well, it's hardly the first treatment one would use.

TC: That's right. It's the kind of approach that disturbs me.

HLN: When you consider injecting mold products like penicillin into people, that doesn't sound very tasteful or logical either.

TC: You're right, but the injection of penicillin is presented to the young doctor in a totally different kind of concept. What I'm saying is that I'm a great believer that you must not shut your mind to new approaches, but I do think you must present new approaches to treatment in an accepted scientific manner for them to be credible.

HLN: That's one of the problems we clinicians

have. I know which techniques work and which don't work, but it would be difficult for me to convince another doctor to understand my work. He would have to sit with me in my office for several weeks, and that's not practical for most physicians.

TC: I think a lot of people were shocked that I didn't hold up a certain interview when I was Assistant Secretary [of the Department of Health, Education and Welfare]. I publicly stated that I took vitamin C after the agency had just given out a big report on this matter that differed with my statement. In fact, the publisher of the newspaper telephoned me to ask if I really said that. I told him I wouldn't say it if I didn't believe it.

HLN: You're a very secure man.

TC: My own personal opinion is not government policy, otherwise there would be a lot of other governmental policies closer to my opinion. It should work both ways.

But I believe that if medical students did get a chance to see firsthand some of these nutritional treatments presented in a logical and scientific manner, they would be receptive to them. When medical students see a physician catheterize a patient because of a heart murmur and the students are given an explanation, then they come to believe it's the right thing to do.

HLN: Right.

TC: But, of course, you can't just send medical students out around the countryside to pick up eclectic experiences. For one thing, there just isn't enough time for that kind of education.

HLN: Is there any particular word you would like to get to the public, any special views?

TC: I recently testified for Senator McGovern's commission again. It's my view that there are great benefits for the public through nutrition throughout society and in the medical profession, in all health professions. I think we need a good program of education. We shouldn't try to approach this by regulation. You do it by education. There are great opportunities in school education programs and in professional-school educational programs. We should use the fantastic tools of communication—like the electronic media—to capture the minds of the public. Important issues like nutrition should not be presented through advertising, not with exposés, but through straight informational material that the public could not get confused about.

In addition, I think that it is quite clear that there are several current American killers—the chronic diseases—where good nutritional therapy in the management of those diseases is greatly underestimated and needs to be put on a par with other treatments.

HLN: Including cancer?

TC: Yes, certainly including the prevention and treatment of cancer.

Dr. Cooper isn't the only one who believes patients with cancer should have better nutrition. Dr. George Blackburn, a surgeon who teaches at Harvard, recently spoke on the subject at a medical meeting in Seattle. His remarks were reported by Jane Brady in *The New York Times* on July 1, 1978.

MALNUTRITION AND SOME DEATHS BY CANCER
ARE LINKED

SEATTLE, June 30—One in 10 * deaths among cancer patients is caused by malnutrition, not by the disease, yet fewer than 1 percent of these patients receive intensive nutritional therapy as part of their treatment, a leading researcher said here today.

Dr. George Blackburn, a surgeon at Harvard Medical School, said that if the cancer patient is well nourished, he can better withstand the side effects of anti-cancer therapy and his body can more effectively fight the cancer and infections that threaten his life. Half to two-thirds of all patients lose a significant amount of weight as a result of cancer, of treatment or both.

---

* I talked with Dr. Blackburn about this figure. He says he was being conservative. Personally I think the figures should be switched to, say 9 in 10.—H.L.N.

Dr. Blackburn was among more than a dozen specialists who cited the importance of good nutrition for cancer patients and who outlined a variety of techniques, including intravenous feeding, for helping patients maintain nutritional well-being. They spoke at a National Conference on Nutrition in Cancer, sponsored by the National Cancer Institute and the American Cancer Society.

Without special nutritional support, Dr. Blackburn said in an interview, the side effects of anti-cancer treatment curtail the patient's chances of overcoming his disease. Although nutritional therapy has not yet been proved to extend the lives of cancer patients or to increase their chances of being cured, Dr. Blackburn said that it greatly improves their quality of life.

"Instead of being bedridden, well-nourished patients are able to get about," he said. "They look good and feel good. The progressive emaciation and dwindling death so common among terminal cancer patients is averted. When they die, they die quickly and less painfully."

Dr. Blackburn cited preliminary data indicating that good nutrition may also improve the patient's chances for survival. In one study, patients who received intensive nutritional therapy were more likely to maintain their natural ability to fight disease, called immunocompetence. One of the consequences of chronic malnutrition is a loss of immunocompetence, Dr. Blackburn said.

Ordinarily, however, only the occasional patient who complains of eating problems gets nutritional support, according to Johanna Dwyer, a nutritionist at the New England Medical Center in Boston.

Among the causes of malnutrition among cancer patients, said Dr. Robert M. Filler, a surgeon at the Hospital for Sick Children in Toronto, are a loss of appetite, changes in taste, the trapping of essential nutrients by the growing cancer, mechanical obstruction of the digestive tract, and the side effects of treatment, such as nausea, vomiting and painful mouth sores.

To counter such effects, a variety of special nutritional techniques are available. According to conference participants, techniques include guidance on the kinds of foods that may be tolerable; the use of special nutritional supplements that can be taken between meals.

17

Diet

If following a diet and taking half a handful of vitamins and minerals several times a day is just not your thing, then forget about this chapter. Take your 10 grams of ascorbic acid a day and expect to have about the same statistical results Cameron and Pauling got in Scotland.

You already know from reading Chapter 1 that a patient with terminal cancer can have his life extended by a factor of four simply by taking 10 grams daily of vitamin C. The research has been done. You have only to turn to the Appendices at the end of this book to see the evidence for that.

The patients in Cameron and Pauling's experiment were given no special dietary instructions, meaning they had the average Scottish diet (which, if anything, is even worse than the average American diet).

But remember that every doctor I have talked with who deals with the nutritional aspects of cancer has the feeling that over-all good nutrition is very important in the battle against cancer. We can't prove our stand, but we all think that Cameron and Pauling would have had better survival rates if they had paid more attention to diet and had given other nutritional supplements along with the vitamin C.

They think so, too.

If it is true that the body's general resistance against cancer is important, then chances are you can improve your odds against beating cancer (and preventing it) if you follow a proper diet.

I can't prove this to you.

If you like, wait a hundred years until scientists can give you a definitive answer. I can only say that a diet that is not biologically stressful is the one I prefer for my patients and the one I select for myself. In my judgment, this is the correct diet for most people fighting cancer, if they take what I consider to be adequate amounts of vitamins and minerals.

There are a few things that scientists have to say regarding cancer and diet:

First: Laboratory animals fed diets low in total calories live longer and develop less cancer.

Second: People who are overweight have an increased incidence of certain cancers—cancer of the breast, for example.

Third: Those who eat a diet high in animal fat and animal protein may have an increased incidence of breast and gastrointestinal cancer.[1]

Fourth: When people have a high intake of fresh fruits (vitamin C) they have a lower over-all incidence of cancer.[2]

Fifth: Laboratory animals can be protected against cancer by being given various vitamins and minerals.

BOY, DOES THAT LEAVE ME CONFUSED!

Certainly you are confused at this point. But now I'm going to sort it all out for you. First let me fill you in on a little ancient history.

Some three to ten million years ago our ancient ancestors lived mainly off fruit in the African jungle. When a severe drought began destroying the forests, our ancestors chose to abandon their habitat and take to the open fields to seek a better source of food. That was when they changed from being fruit eaters to hunters and meat eaters.

For at least three million years our ancestors lived chiefly off meat. Only during the past five to ten thousand years has man turned into an agricultural animal and made grains (using wheat products such as bread and pasta in the West and rice in the East) and milk (and products made of milk such as cheese) a part of his diet. Sugar has been in our diet in significant amounts for less than two hundred years.

The biochemistry of our bodies had three million years to adapt itself to meat eating. Those of our ancestors who could not eat meat and thrive simply died off and did not reproduce. By natural selection, our ancestors were adapted to meat eating.

Nature has only five to ten thousand years to adapt us to grains and milk, and a mere two hundred years to adapt us to sugar.

It is simply not possible to wipe out three million years of natural selection in a mere ten thousand years.

This Will Help Make It Clearer

We are all aware that each animal has its own natural diet. If you had a prize rabbit, for example, you wouldn't try to raise it on beefsteak. If you owned a million-dollar racehorse you wouldn't feed it oat-flavored hamburgers.

Let's have a closer look at the horse.

If you decided to change horses from grain-eating animals to meat-eating animals, you would first round up a large collection of horses and start them on their new diets.

You would find some of the horses wouldn't eat hamburger no matter how much rye flavor you added. They wouldn't eat the hamburgers even if you made them into small pellets that resembled rye.

These horses you would set aside as worthless for your experiment, and you would turn your attention to the horses that would eat the new diet. You would observe them to see how they fared on the hamburger-flavored rye.

Some of them would lie around on the grass exhausted and half sick from the new diet. Others would have headaches or gas or constipation or diarrhea. One or two of the horses might do fairly well on the new diet. They might not be smiling and running to the trough when you came to feed them, but at least they would be on their feet and halfway functioning.

These few horses would be the ones you would keep for your experiment. You would breed them together, and then you would breed those of their offspring that did best on beef, and so on and on, selectively breeding your horses through the years, through the centuries and millennia. It would take an extraordinarily long time before such selective breeding would produce a horse that could really thrive on beef and outrun the old-fashioned grain-eating horse. It takes a very long time for nature to establish a breed of animal that can thrive on a new diet.

That's why meat is still the natural diet for mankind.

We can function on a diet of grain and milk and sugar, but most people (I did not say everyone) function best on a high-meat diet. It is usually the diet best suited for our biochemistry.

It is the diet which is the least stressful for the most people. Remember the word *stressful* because we will be returning to it shortly.

HOW DO WE KNOW MEAT IS MAN'S NATURAL DIET?

First, we have anthropological evidence that meat is our most ancient food. Every ancient living site inhabited by our ancestors has been strewn with bones of animals killed for food.

Anthropologists have also learned a great deal about the diet of ancient man by studying the stomach contents of bog bodies (bodies that have been preserved in bogs). They have also examined coprolites (dessicated or petrified feces) in microscopic detail, which give much information about the food eaten.

Although mankind has had fire for some three hundred thousand years, it did not become popular until about fifty thousand years ago. The oldest pottery discovered—and remember, pottery is very easily preserved—comes from Catal Huyuk, Turkey, and dates back only seven thousand years. Without the use of fire and pottery, modern foods such as wheat and other grains, potatoes, and beans would have been absent from the diet.

We can conclude that any food which cannot be digested without first being cooked is unnatural to man; that he has not yet had enough time for his enzyme systems to become efficient in handling that food; and that that food is stressful for him.

Second, our ancient ancestors, the ones who were still living in the forests and eating primarily fruit, had very large flat molars, almost as large as quarters. Such teeth were designed to chew vegetables and fruit. Our teeth have been evolving toward those of a meat eater, with smaller molar surfaces. Had grain not come into our diet a few thousand years ago, in all probability our teeth would have continued their evolutionary trend toward sharpness, so that eventually they would have ended up much like those of a cat or dog. We lost our fangs because man did not need fangs for killing. We are a weapon-using creature and carry our fangs in our hands.

Third, I have an unending stream of sick patients consulting me. Perhaps not deadly sick, but less than well. These people are suffering from high blood pressure, constipation, degenerative heart diseases, arthritis, diabetes, tiredness, depression, obesity, dermatitis, anxiety, and a host of other disorders to which mankind is heir. Most of these people have been on a diet heavy in the "new" foods, foods which have come along with the advent of civilization, such as grains, milk products, and sweets. Once patients are taken off these "new" foods and placed on more primitive diets heavy on animal fat and animal protein, light on vegetables and fruits, and entirely free of sugar, grains, and milk and milk products, they very often rapidly lose their complaints.

THE CHOLESTEROL PROBLEM

As all literate people know, the current fashion in diet is running against animal meat and animal fats. Physicians have been seeking to control our national epidemic of coronary artery disease (and other vascular degenerative diseases) by reducing cholesterol in the daily diet.

I am convinced that reducing meat and animal fat in the diet is the wrong way to go about controlling cholesterol levels and hardening of the arteries.

Allen B. Nichols, M.D., and his associates at the University of Michigan, for example, recently completed an in-depth dietary-cholesterol study of 4,057 adults in the town of Tecumseh, Michigan. The only correlation they found with high cholesterol blood levels was weight.

The people who were overweight had high cholesterol levels. The people who were not overweight had lower cholesterol levels. It made no difference whatsoever what type of diet they were following.*

The following studies have also shown that low-cholesterol diets do not reduce the incidence of heart attacks:

1. The St. Mary's Hospital Trial (1965)
2. The London Research Committee's Trial (1965)
3. The Norwegian Trial (1966)
4. The Anti-Coronary Club Trial (1966)
5. The London Medical Research Council Trial (1968)
6. The National Diet Heart Study (1968)
7. The Finnish Mental Hospital Trial (1968)
8. The Los Angeles Veterans' Trial (1969)
9. The Farmingham Study (1970)
10. The Ireland-Boston Heart Study (1970)

---

* You can read a report of these findings in the conservative *Journal of the American Medical Association,* vol. 236 (1976), p. 17.

11. The St. Vincent's Hospital Trial (1973)
12. The Diet and Coronary Heart Disease Study in England (1974)
13. The Edinburgh-Stockholm Study (1975)
14. The Minnesota Study (1975)
15. The UCLA Study (1975)
16. The Honolulu-Japanese Study (1975)

In addition, the Coronary Drug Project (1974) showed that reducing serum cholesterol levels by the use of medication did not lower the incidence of heart disease.

Many of the men who have championed the low-cholesterol diet for heart protection have been in teaching positions or in public health. They have not been earning their living in a one-to-one doctoring relationship with patients.

Having sustained a coronary myself some twelve years ago, I have a very personal interest in the prevention of heart disease. In fact, my life depends upon making the right decisions about whether or not to eat meat and animal fats.

Dr. Richard Passwater, in his interesting book *Supernutrition for Healthy Hearts,* makes an interesting offer:

> No one has ever shown that eating cholesterol causes heart disease. If anyone can step forward and prove that eating cholesterol causes heart disease, I will donate my proceeds from this book to the American Heart Association.[3]

PATIENT EXAMPLE

Recently a dentist who had been to Cleveland Clinic for bypass coronary artery surgery consulted me. They had sent him home on the usual low-cholesterol, low-meat, low-animal-fat diet. When I tested him, his HDL was 30!

HDL is the medical jargon for high-density lipoproteins. It has been well established that coronary artery disease is much more closely associated with HDL levels than with cholesterol levels. The higher the HDL figure, the less likely the patient is to have a coronary. When it gets down into the 30s you worry. This patient's HDL lacked only one point of being in the 20s.

I placed him on a high-fat, high-animal-protein, low-carbohydrate diet as well as on nutritional supplements, including 26 grams of vitamin C (a great cholesterol lowerer and HDL elevator) daily. After six weeks on this program his HDL had risen to 46!

I eat a high-animal-fat, high-meat diet and my HDL is 67.

I could cite hundreds of similar patients under my care.

I know from personal experience how to handle the coronary artery problem: Most people do very well on a high-meat, high-animal-fat diet *if* they take the proper supplements.

The key to keeping cholesterol levels down and HDL levels up is nutritional supplements: especially vitamin C, vitamin B_6, the entire B complex, dolomite, lecithin, safflower oil, and sometimes niacin (one form of vitamin B_3).

BUT ISN'T MEAT CONTAMINATED WITH HORMONES AND ANTIBIOTICS?

My friend, everything on our planet is contaminated at this point in time. Even mother's milk is radioactive and often does not reach the standards required for interstate shipment of cow's milk.

And you think the wheat in your daily bread is not contaminated? It's sprayed with chemicals while it's growing. Once it's in the silo, it's sprayed to keep out the insects, sprayed again to repel rats, and shot full of chemicals to retard mold. After it goes to the man who makes your packaged bread and cookies, it is often sprayed a few more times.

As if this were not contamination enough, the Department of Agriculture allows an *average* of two rat-dropping pellets per quart of wheat. If you're unlucky some morning and the dice haven't fallen just right for you, you may well have four rat pellets in your sweet roll!

Gives you something to think about, doesn't it?

I won't go into sugar and milk. Believe me, they have their problems too.

WYNDER'S VIEWS

One of the chief advocates for the use of a low-meat, low-animal-fat diet for the avoidance of cancer and cardiovascular disease is Ernst L. Wynder, M.D., President of the American Health Foundation, who was good enough to have me in for an interview so I could hear his arguments firsthand.

In reviewing the tape I made of our conversation, I found that Wynder wanted to make several points against the meat and animal-fat diet:

A diet heavy in meat (with its accompanying animal fat), Dr. Wynder said, *is unnatural to man. Our ancestors were vegetarians.*

Let me say that I think this view of Wynder's is entirely false. Robert Ardrey's wonderful book *The Hunting Hypothesis* [4] and the Brothwells in their *Food in Antiquity* [5] both conclude that ancient man's diet was made up primarily of meat and animal fat. I have discussed this point with Dr. Glenn Conroy (who, incidentally, is a heavy meat eater himself) of the Department of Anthropology at New York University. He agrees with the sources cited.

Wild game, Dr. Wynder pointed out, *has very little fat compared with the marbelized fat that we see on feedlot cattle slaughtered in this country.*

True. You will agree if you've ever eaten venison. But deer, as well as the ibex, bison, and horse (which constituted the greatest part of man's diet in antiquity) does have fat on it. Most of the fat is located in a layer just underneath the skin. When we kill a deer and skin it, most of the fat is thrown away with the skin. Undoubtedly, primitive man did not waste hard-earned food. He carefully scraped the fat off and ate it along with the meat. Also, he got a generous amount of fat when he ate the liver and the brains of these animals.

I have already stated why I conclude meat and animal fats are man's natural diet. Man has not been a vegetarian for millions of years. I and every source I have contacted disagree with Wynder's views.

Wynder says he believes *a heavy meat diet (and the fat that comes with it) causes heart attacks.* I have already discussed the fallacy of this view.

Wynder states that *a high-carbohydrate diet will not make people fat if they are properly instructed about eating habits.*

I made the point with Dr. Wynder that if people didn't get their calories from meat (and the fat that accompanies it), they would get fat, because all they would have left to eat would be carbohydrates.

You cannot devise a diet without meat, fat, or carbohydrates, because you end up with only air on your plate.

It has been well known for more than a century— William Banting, a London mortician, published a pamphlet on this subject in 1864—that people get fat by eating carbohydrates, not by eating meat.

The bases of the most successful weight-reduction diets have been proteins and fats. Check out the Stillman or the Atkins diets. I have been interested in weight reduction for a number of years and have written a book on the subject, *Dr. Newbold's Revolutionary New Discoveries About Weight Loss.* I have struggled with patients who want to lose weight long enough to know what will make the pounds go away and what will not.

Eating carbohydrates will not make them lose weight for one simple reason: People cannot control their appetites when eating carbohydrates. At least 40 percent of our population will be overweight if they eat carbohydrates in significant amounts.

These same people can control their appetites if they eat meat and fats. They will not be fat on such a diet.

Dr. Wynder's argument was that people simply need to be trained through behavioral conditioning to eat properly, to eat carbohydrates in moderation, and then they won't be fat.

I venture to say that if Dr. Wynder tried to earn his living teaching people to eat carbohydrates in moderation with behavioral techniques, he would soon be buying his food and paying his rent with checks issued by the New York Department of Human Resources.

Brother, it won't work. I know—I've been there, both as a doctor who helps patients lose weight and as a former fatty myself.

I asked Dr. Robert Atkins what he thought of Wynder's plan to have people control their appetites with behavioral conditioning while eating diets high in carbohydrates. He scoffed at the idea: unrealistic pipe dreams from the ivory tower.

I say to you loud and clear: *Forty percent of you will be overweight if you follow a high-carbohydrate diet.*

That 40 percent will have an increased death rate from high blood pressure, heart disease, stroke, accidents, diabetes, and, yes, even cancer, because certain forms of cancer (breast cancer in women, for example) are found more frequently in fat people than in slender people.

Japanese women, Dr. Wynder pointed out, *have a low incidence of breast cancer in Japan (where they are said to eat a low-meat, low-fat diet) but have a higher rate of breast cancer when they move to Hawaii (where they are said to have a high-meat, high-fat diet).*

Even the casual reader will realize that there are vast differences between the women's environment in Japan and in Hawaii.

First, we must know how the meat and fat were cooked in the two countries. It is well known that browned meat (as usually prepared in the West) gives a positive Ames test, which means that it is mutagenic and probably carcinogenic. Does this risk limit itself only to the gastrointestinal tract, or could other organs such as the breast also be involved? At least 90 percent of the population has whole, undigested particles of protein absorbed directly into the bloodstream from the gut. Why should the singed portions of meat be excluded from this process?

The second factor that should be taken into consideration is the fuel used to cook the meat and fat, since foods absorb particles of the fuels to which they are exposed. For example, many of my allergic patients do not tolerate meat broiled under a gas flame, whereas they may eat meat without having a reaction if it is broiled under electric heat. To me this means meat broiled under gas absorbs hydrocarbons from the gas flame. It is well known that hydrocarbons are carcinogenic. I suspect that meat and animal fat are often blamed for sins which in reality are committed by the gas company.

I might add in passing that I find many allergic patients have intolerances to browned meat and animal fat. If they eat the same meat boiled or pressure-cooked (the methods which experience has taught me to recommend) then they may eat the meat in perfect safety.

Even the cut of meat may be important for allergic individuals, indicating that different parts of the carcass are chemically different and hence may well have different effects upon the person eating it.

We think of rib roast as simply being more tender than chuck steak, for example. But if you will boil each of these cuts in separate pans and taste them without adding seasoning, you will understand at once that their flavors are quite different, indicating a chemical difference between the two cuts. I find many of my patients can tolerate rib steaks when they cannot tolerate (from an allergic standpoint) chuck steak. Do different cuts of meat also have different effects on cancer rates?

Even the feed an animal eats will change the flavor

of the meat, its allergenicity, and hence its chemistry and possibly its effect on cancer rates.

So when we speak of meat and animal fat, we are lumping many factors together which must be separated if we are to talk intelligently about the carcinogenic propensities of meat.

But the problem is more complicated yet.

In Chapter 20 I point out the rather convincing evidence that vitamin E gives laboratory animals protection against carcinogenic chemicals. It is well accepted the added unsaturated fat calls for additional amounts of vitamin E. It follows, then, that statistical studies are meaningless unless the subjects under consideration have been tested for serum vitamin E levels.

And what about other vitamins and minerals that I mentioned in the chapter on the prevention of cancer by the use of nutrients? How can epidemiological studies have any meaning if the vitamin A and B levels are not studied, along with the vitamin C levels, the selenium levels, and the zinc levels?

And what about processed meats and fats that contain preservatives (like nitrates), food coloring, and other chemicals. What about the amount of sugar eaten? What about the relative change in weight?

Quite obviously, figures that talk about high-meat diets causing cancer are ridiculous. They simply play into the popular misconceptions about meat that basically all go back to mankind's reluctance to admit that he has been a professional killer and has lived off his kill for at least three million years. "Scientists" still haven't got around to accepting Darwin's ideas, which are a hundred years old.

Interestingly enough, Denis Burkitt has made a great deal out of the importance of roughage in speeding up the total time food spends in the body. We must remember that fats also speed up passage time.

Of course, Linus Pauling maintains that it makes no difference what you eat so long as you take adequate amounts of vitamin C.[6]

We must not forget that it is in the parts of Africa

and Asia where animal proteins are in inadequate supply that we find more cancer of the liver.

Dr. Good in Chapter 14 has noted the frequency with which cancer appears among people suffering from kwashiorkor, a nutritional deficiency disease.

So What Can We Eat?

Both historical facts and my clinical experience lead me to believe that the average wheat-heavy, sugar-heavy, milk and milk-products-heavy American diet that contains processed foods is stressful for most people.

If we work on the theory that the human body can fight off disease (including cancer) better if it is not under biochemical stress, then it makes sense to eat the kind of caveman diet our enzyme systems were designed by nature to handle.

In my judgment, the ideal diet for people who want to avoid cancer and for patients engaged in a battle against cancer would be:

1. All the fresh meat, fresh fowl, fresh seafood desired. *These should be steamed, boiled, or pressure-cooked.* In order to keep an adequate intake of calories, one must eat enough of the fat to satisfy the appetite.* Animal protein and fat should be the backbone of the diet. Meat should be cooked rare.

2. Modest amounts of fresh vegetables, raw or lightly steamed.

3. Modest amounts of fresh fruit. By modest I mean one piece of fruit, as dessert, after each meal.

4. Avoidance of all processed foods, such as canned foods, dried foods, frozen foods, made-up foods such as hot dogs and salami.

5. Drinking only spring water bottled in glass or water you boil for ten minutes and then distill yourself in a stainless-steel distiller and store in glass bottles. If

---

* Your vitamin C and other supplements will keep your cholesterol down.

you buy spring water that has been bottled in plastic, pour it into a wide-mouth container and let it sit for twenty-four hours so the gases from the plastic can escape. Do not buy bottled distilled water. For some reason I do not understand, it often disagrees with people.

Note well: My advice about diet and water is valid only if you are taking vitamins and minerals as recommended by me.

18

Feeding the Terminally Ill Patient

A few months ago I was called to see a dying cancer patient at one of New York's leading teaching hospitals. One end of the old man's bed was raised. The poor bag of bones was so weak that he was slumped down into a half-sitting position and would have fallen out of the bed entirely if it had not been for the side rails. A plastic tube was taped to his cheek. It ran down his nose to his stomach. Although he had met me a few years previously, when I had treated another member of the family, his eyes were blank as he looked my way. A few questions revealed he didn't know who he was, where he was, or what was happening to him.

Obviously this patient was near death. The tube feeding was causing most of his stupor and certainly was contributing to his poor condition.

I looked at the white liquid that slid down the tube into his stomach. This was one of those "scientific" formulas put out by several drug companies to supply "total nutrition" to patients who were unable to take food by mouth. I have checked out their formulas: They are usually made with amino acids (chemically broken down protein), milk solids, corn syrup, some fat, plus a few synthetic vitamins and minerals. At my last count there were eighteen of these formulas on the market.

If you want to get bombed out of your head some weekend, take a few bottles of these mixtures home with you on Friday night and drink it in place of food for a couple of days.

FOOD ALLERGIES

We tend to think of allergies as consisting only of such ailments as hay fever, hives, or asthma. We tend to forget that the central nervous system can also be involved in allergic reactions. We can have different shock organs involved during an allergic attack. If the nose is the shock organ, we have hay fever or rhinitis. If the skin is the shock organ, we have hives or eczema. If the lungs are the shock organ, we develop asthma.

But the brain can also be the shock organ, in which case we may experience depression, tiredness, restlessness, hallucinations, or confusion, to name only a few possible symptoms.

The "scientific" food mixtures such as the patient was receiving are fairly well made from a theoretical standpoint: They may be adequate in basic calories, protein, vitamins (but not the crude source that we also need), and a few of the more important minerals. But these mixtures have been supervised by men who are not intimately familiar with the importance of food allergies, hence the allergic aspects of nutrition have been neglected.

Many people might eat the kind of foods included in these pseudo-scientific formulas without having any reaction. Many others, however, will experience reactions, especially people in poor health, when their brains are already somewhat toxic from illness.

NATURAL VERSUS SYNTHETIC

Roger Williams, Professor Emeritus of Biochemistry at the University of Texas, has pointed out in his wonderful book *Nutrition Against Disease* that unknown factors are needed for proper nutrition. When attempts are made to grow human tissue artificially in a nutrient broth, scientists fail unless they add a small amount of human serum, which contains the unknown factors needed by the tissue.

Dr. William R. Murphy, who received a Nobel prize for discovering that injections of liver extract would control pernicious anemia, told me that he believes there are as-yet-undiscovered nutrients needed by the human body. As an example, he cites an experience from his own practice. When purified vitamin B_{12} came along in the late 1940s, he tried switching his pernicious anemia patients to that product. Even though the purified vitamin controlled their anemia, many of the patients did not feel as good as when they were given the crude form of the vitamin in crude-liver injections.

Albert Szent-Györgyi, who received a Nobel prize for discovering vitamin C, has told me he thinks vitamin C must have certain unknown factors to work with to be effective.

Recently I talked with Richard Edward Auslic, Associate Professor of Animal Nutrition at Cornell University. His research is in agreement with that of the other authorities I have cited: Humans must have as-yet-unidentified nutrients in their diet.

Patients are not going to get these unidentified substances in the "scientific" formulas mentioned.

In summary, the formulas should not be fed to patients for two reasons: They contain highly allergenic foods and they are not a complete food.

MY FORMULA

I'm afraid no drug company is going to get rich off the formula I suggest, because it can be made from common foods from your neighborhood grocery store, using utensils that can be bought in most department stores. This formula could easily be made up by hospital dieticians, but I will be willing to bet it won't be. It's much easier to open a can than to prepare a meal.

You'll have to make my formula at home and carry it to the hospital, if that is where your loved one happens to be. Of course, you must get his doctor's approval.

Here are the steps. Anyone can follow them:

1. Buy a fresh, unaged 1-pound steak. People are much more likely to react allergically to aged meat.

Be careful about the butcher. I find they are often not very honest about their products. Do not ask: "Have you any unaged steak?" He would probably give you the answer most likely to put cash into his pocket. (I have nothing against butchers. I am simply reporting experiences I have had with them.)

Instead, ask: "Are all your steaks aged?" He will probably say yes with great pride and accidentally tell you the truth.

In general, prime, *unsalted* kosher rib steaks are best for the present purpose, because religious laws forbid the aging of kosher meat. Do not buy frozen kosher (or any other) steaks.

In the West and Midwest you can often buy good fresh beef at chain grocery stores. I haven't had very good luck with chain-store beef here in New York.

Look at the steak to make sure it is soft and bright red, not the duller red that appears when meat is aged. If you buy it from a chain store, go early in the morning and wait while they cut your steak. Give them a piece of aluminum foil to wrap it in. Have them put the dull side of the foil against the steak. Avoid plastic wrappings. What is today called butcher's wax paper is often plastic-impregnated.

2. Cut off any of the blue stamping that might remain (but leave most of the fat) and place the steak in a stainless-steel pressure cooker. If it's a 4-quart cooker, add ½ cup bottled-in-glass spring water.

Bring it up to full pressure and let it cook there for about forty minutes.* When you remove the steak, it

---

* Some patients do better on rare meat. Try both rare and well done.

should be quite soft, so soft you can pull it apart with two forks.

Shred the steak with two forks. Place the short shreds in an ordinary blender, add 2 glasses of bottled-in-glass spring water, turn the blender on high, and leave it there for about five minutes.

The result will be a very fine liquid steak (including the fat), which will be the mainstay of the diet. It should be fine enough to go down a stomach tube.

Note: If you live in South America or in a part of Europe or another place where the cattle are range-fed (rather than feedlot-fed) the meat may have too little fat on it. In that case you will need to add some beef brains to the steak in order to give it more fat. We cannot live on lean meat alone. I suggest about 1 slightly rounded tablespoon of calf brain to 1 pound of lean meat.

Your steak mixture should be refrigerated in a glass container at once. Any unused portion should be discarded at the end of the day, because, as every housewife knows, ground meat ages faster than whole meat.

VEGETABLES

Vegetables should be prepared separately, one at a time. Only fresh vegetables should be used. These must be washed with soap* and warm water. The following is a list of allowed vegetables.

Asparagus	Cauliflower
Beet greens	Celery
Broccoli	Chard
Brussels sprouts	Chicory
Cabbage	Collards
Carrots	Cucumber

---

* Rokeach soap is best. It's available in many grocery stores in Jewish neighborhoods.

Dandelions	Pepper, green
Escarole	Poke
Kale	Romaine lettuce
Lettuce	Spinach
Mustard greens	Summer squash
Okra	Turnip greens
Parsley	Watercress

Place a cup of vegetables on a cutting board and chop it finely. Then place it in a blender, add ½ cup water, and turn blender on high for about five minutes.

Remove and store in refrigerator in a glass container. Keep no longer than one day.

FRUITS

This is a list of allowed *fresh* fruits:

Apple	Honeydew melon
Apricot	Orange
Banana	Peach
Berries	Pear
Cherries	Plum
Cranshaw melon	Strawberry
Grapefruit	Tangerine
Grapes	

Wash and if possible skin fruit. Place 1 cup of the diced fruit in the blender. Add ½ cup water. Turn blender on high for five minutes. If the mixture is too thick, add another ½ cup water and mix again briefly.

You now have one day's food: steak, vegetable, and fruit.

Changing from one form of food to another is a somewhat tricky business, since the body must make multiple adjustments. Most of these adjustments (such as change in the bacterial flora of the gut) can take place in a week, but other more subtle adjustments may require a month. *Do not,* I repeat, *do not suddenly* switch a patient who has been on artificial food for as long as several days to the foods mentioned here. If you do switch suddenly you may cause unpleasant side effects such as nausea and diarrhea.

I would suggest that no more than ½ cup of the meat mixture and ¼ cup of either the vegetable or the fruit mixture be given for the first meal. (Remember, we are talking about tube-feeding meals.) The amount of the hospital's artificial tube-feeding formula should be cut in half. The mixture which you have made at home should be heated to body temperature just before it is administered.

The mixture you make at home should be fed only once the first day, twice the second day, and three times the third day. If at the end of three days the mixture is being well accepted, then the hospital mixture should be gradually phased out and your mixture gradually increased until it constitutes the patient's entire diet.

THE NEXT STEP

Once the decision has been made to give nutritional support to the cancer patient, several things must be done at once.

First step: Collect two heaping tablespoons of hair from the head. This should be taken from several different spots, cut close to the scalp in the back of the head. The first two inches of hair should be used; any that is longer than that should be cut off and thrown away. The patient's physician should send the hair sample to: Parmae Laboratories, P.O. Box 35227, Airlawn Station, Dallas, Texas 75235.

He should make a request for a "Profile 1," which will give an analysis of seventeen trace minerals, including toxic minerals such as lead and arsenic.

Only by having a mineral survey will it be possible to make final decision about what minerals to give the patient. For many reasons, the sodium- and potassium-level reports on hair tests are not usually very reliable and should be ignored.

Second step: Have the patient's physician administer hydroxocobalamin (vitamin B_{12b}), 500 micrograms by intramuscular injection. If this seems to give the patient a lift, 1,000 micrograms should be injected on the next day. If the lift comes again, then the patient may need this injection daily, or even two or three times a day, depending upon how long the lift continues. In any case, the vitamin should be given frequently enough so that it does not give a lift. If the patient continues to get a lift from each injection, then the injections are being spaced too far apart.

Think of the diabetic. You would not wait until the diabetic's blood sugar was out of control and making him sick before giving an injection of insulin. The injection should be given *before* it is needed, not after. So with vitamin B_{12b}.

Third Step: Have the physician inject 0.25 milliliter of crude liver extract the first day, 0.5 milliliter the second day, 1 milliliter the third, and then continue with 1 milliliter three times a week.

ADD THESE VITAMINS

The meat blend you made should be fed four times a day after the patient gets past the first few days on the new diet. After the patient has been getting some of the mixture for three days, start adding vitamins to the mixture (blend them into the food with the blender) as follows:

1. Take a gelatin pearl containing 10,000 units of natural vitamin A and 400 units of natural vitamin D and puncture it with a pin. Squeeze the contents into the meat mixture that will be fed at breakfast. Add this amount again at the evening meal.

2. Take a gelatin pearl containing 200 units of alpha-tocopherol acetate, puncture it with a pin, and squeeze the contents into the breakfast meal only.

3. Pull apart a Hy B Complex 50 capsule. Mix ¼ of the powder from this capsule into the breakfast and supper feedings.

4. Buy some sugar-free, starch-free folic acid tablets, 1 milligram each. (This will require a prescription.) Crush 2 tablets and blend them in with the food four times a day.

5. Add ¼ teaspoon citrus bioflavonoid powder to breakfast and supper feedings.

6. Buy a bottle of safflower oil that has no preservative in it (that which you buy in grocery stores usually contains a preservative; try a health food store and read the label) and add ¼ teaspoon to each of the four daily feedings. Refrigerate unused oil.

7. Blend lecithin into the food you have prepared. If you use the lecithin granules, add 1 heaping teaspoon to each feeding and gradually, over the course of ten days, increase this to 2 heaping teaspoons at each feeding. If you use liquid lecithin, halve the amount. Lecithin should be refrigerated after opening.

8. Add ½ teaspoon of either brewer's or primary yeast to the food mixture morning and night. Gradually over a two-week period increase to 1 teaspoon at each of the four feedings.

MINERALS

Don't forget to order the hair test mentioned previously. It will help in planning exactly which mineral to give.

While you are waiting for the results of the hair test, start the following minerals.

1. Dolomite powder, ¼ teaspoon in each of the four feedings.

2. Zinc gluconate. To administer, pull apart a 60 milligram capsule and add the contents to three of the daily feedings.

3. Crush 1 kelp tablet, blend it in well with the food mixture, and add to one feeding daily.

And so there you have the details for what I believe to be ideal food for the patient who appears to be terminally ill.

He will of course be getting the vitamin C by intravenous injection, as covered in Chapter 22. As soon as possible, cautiously begin adding vitamin C by mouth, but be certain not to give enough to produce gas, upset stomach, or diarrhea.

NOW HEAR THIS WELL

By the time patients have reached the "terminally ill" stage everyone has already crossed him off his list.

"He's suffering so much. He'd be better off dead," you hear the family and doctor say. Or "After all, he's had eighty-one good years. It's his time."

At this point the simple truth is everyone wants the patient dead.

The hospital authorities want to make way for a new patient. (The hospital makes more money on a new patient because new patients have many laboratory and X-ray studies and perhaps operating room fees, all of which help with the overhead.)

It's frustrating to the doctor to have a patient he can't cure.

The family is tired of using up their spare time in visiting the hospitalized patient, of smiling and trying to make conversation with someone they probably haven't had a twenty-minute talk with for a quarter of a century. They think about the money the patient is spending: The more he spends, the less they will inherit. They are already visualizing the new car they're going to get with money left to them in the will.

But don't forget we're talking about human life, the most valuable thing in the world, more valuable than diamonds and gold. In the last analysis, life is all we have. Everyone has a right to as much of it as he can get.

In the Appendix A of this book you will see the paper written by Ewan Cameron and Linus Pauling.

All of the patients they treat with vitamin C were terminally ill. They were started on massive amounts of vitamin C in the early 1970s. Some of them are still well and healthy, going about their daily lives, eating and working and having sex and doing whatever else gives them pleasure and fulfillment.

I once had an eighty-six-year-old patient who everyone thought was terminally ill. Except for me and a devoted daughter, they all wanted to let the man die in peace.

Well, we brought him around. He went home and lived for more than five years. Furthermore, he enjoyed life. He sat in the sun in the park and fed the pigeons, and he went for walks, and he watched the ball games on TV, and he was glad to be alive.

Now I'm going to let you in on a medical secret: If you have a terminally ill relative whom you are determined to save, you'd be better off with a young doctor in private practice. An older, well-established doctor has plenty of patients. A young, hungry doctor is more likely to hang on and work like the devil to save every patient, for two very selfish (but very human) reasons: the longer the patient lives, the more money the doctor will make, and he might not be able to easily replace the patient with another one. Also, if the patient lives when everyone expected him to die, the word will get around. The doctor's small reputation will be expanded. Again, to be crude but honest, it's money in his pocket.

19

How to Stop Smoking

No book on cancer would be complete without a chapter on tobacco smoking, which alone accounts for one third of the cancer deaths of men in this country. The women are rapidly reaching equality, at least in this matter.

It seems extraordinary to me that any government that pretends to have the best interest of its citizens at heart does not do more to discourage the use of tobacco.

The government has soldiers to protect us from invaders, police to protect us from criminals, firemen to protect us from fire, public health service doctors to protect us from illness, the FDA to protect us from harmful foods. Why does the government not only not protect us from tobacco, but actually encourage the use of tobacco by allowing it to be shipped in interstate commerce, by permitting advertisements for it to be carried through the mail, and by actually giving our tax money to tobacco farmers to help them make more off their crops of death?

To allow smoking is unfair to us nonsmokers. For one thing, it takes money out of our pockets.

For example, our tax money, in part, pays for education through governmental support of schools and universities. If I pay for Mr. Y's education and he smokes tobacco, gets lung cancer, and dies at age fifty-three, rather than at age sixty-three, I haven't gotten my money's worth out of my investment in his education.

Worse yet, when he gets cancer he will go to a hospital that is probably supported in part by my tax money. He will receive hospitalization insurance, which means the amount of money I have to pay for my insurance will increase.

It makes me boil to see people smoke. I know every puff they take is costing me money. But, worse still, it is painful for me to watch people throwing away the only thing they really have: life itself.

I've spent most of my years trying to help people get well and live longer. How can I stand idly by and watch them waste what I have fought so hard to help them save?

If we passed a law stripping everyone in this country of all their wealth, taking every penny from every person, there would be marching in the streets, possibly a revolution. People wouldn't stand for it. Yet every day people simply blow away their most valuable possession: life. At this moment I am richer than Howard Hughes, John Paul Getty, and King Faisal of Arabia combined, because I have life and they do not.

CANCER IS ONLY PART OF THE HARM

If cancer were the only harm of tobacco, maybe I could live with that, but it is only one among many of the damages. People who smoke are more prone to cardiovascular disease: Buerger's disease, coronary artery disease, high blood pressure, stroke.

Most people are not aware of the emotional problems stemming from tobacco, but in my office, where we do provocative tests for tobacco allergy, it is quite obvious to us that tobacco is the source of much emotional trouble.

Example: Several months ago, when we tested a young lady, a smoker, for allergy to tobacco, she turned on one of the other patients being tested and wanted to know why she was being stared at. She even tried to provoke an argument with the technician performing the tests.

Of course, I do not maintain that in every instance of paranoia tobacco is the cause, but in some it is. We have seen many other symptoms produced by tobacco: tiredness, abdominal cramps, pain in the hands or legs, nervousness, insomnia, depression, and even confusion and schizophrenic behavior.

All My Patients Must Stop Smoking

I have learned that it is impossible for me to work out a proper diet for a patient so long as he is smoking. Why? Because to get the proper diet I must introduce foods to the body one at a time and let the body, in one way or another, tell me if these foods are suitable for that particular patient. I must ask the questions properly and I must have the body free of symptoms before it can give me clear-cut answers.

If a patient is smoking, the body is confused and cannot give me a clear answer. For this reason, all my patients must stop smoking.

But that's not the only reason. I feel I'm wasting my time with patients who smoke. If they are smoking, they are only playing games. They don't have any real interest in good health. I'd rather save my time for a serious patient.

So, having helped hundreds and perhaps thousands of patients to stop smoking, I am in a position to give some practical advice on the matter.

What Is an Addiction?

The World Health Organization has defined addiction as having these characteristics:

1. An overpowering desire or need (compulsion) to continue taking the drug and to obtain it by any means.

2. A tendency to increase the dose.

3. A psychic (psychological) and sometimes a physical dependency on the effects of the drug.

If you take away the word *drug* and substitute the word *tobacco* you have an excellent description of tobacco addiction.

A few years ago, a group of scientists at Japan's Kyoto University did a laboratory study of addiction. They grew chick embryo tissue in a nutrient soup and then added morphine to the soup for a number of weeks until the tissue was "addicted."

The next step was to stop adding the morphine. When they did this, the embyro tissue stopped growing.

Under the microscope the cells showed signs of physical degeneration: They were twisted and shrunken, and their nuclei were misshapen.

As the final step in the experiment, morphine was once more added to the nutrient soup, after which the cells started growing again. Now, under the microscope, the cells showed a normal, healthy appearance. They were once more fat and undistorted.

This experiment led to the conclusion that addictive substances, like morphine, become so incorporated into the metabolic chemistry of the cells that when such substances are withdrawn the cells' internal chemistry is completely disrupted.

Tobacco Is an Addictive Substance

We are surrounded in our society by addictive substances, chemicals to which we become accustomed, to the point where we experience withdrawal symptoms if we don't get them regularly. Everyone knows that narcotics such as codeine, morphine, and heroin are addictive subtances, but many people are not fully aware that things like coffee, sugar, wheat products, alcoholic drinks, and tobacco are equally addictive. Vast industries in this country are founded upon the financially solid rock of addiction.

Ask any smoker who has given up the habit and

he will tell you he felt restless, nervous, depressed, unsatisfied, belligerent, and had a craving for sweets when he gave up tobacco.

(Man, you will remember, craved sweets because he was under stress. Before the arrival of table sugar, the craving was satisfied with fruits, which was nature's way of providing him with extra amounts of ascorbic acid during times of stress.)

The symptoms which the smoker experiences when he leaves off the weed are due to withdrawal. His body cells have incorporated chemicals from tobacco into their metabolism. When these chemicals are suddenly taken away, the cellular chemistry is temporarily disrupted. This results in the symptoms listed.

The worst of the withdrawal symptoms occur during the first five days. Usually the third day is the bleakest.

After the acute withdrawal stage there comes a much longer period during which the body has a strong "memory" for the joys of smoking.

For a year or two after I gave up cigars I liked to sit downwind from a cigar smoker and enjoy some of the smoke that wafted my way. Now, after many years, I simply find the smell of smoke annoying.

How to Stop Smoking

You've heard about different methods to stop smoking: filters that can be twisted a notch each day so that by the end of two weeks you are smoking mostly air; drugs that are supposed to curb your desire to smoke; group programs where smokers first learn all the reasons they should stop smoking and are then instructed to cut down one or two cigarettes a day until they're free of the habit; or perhaps your cocktail-party friends talk about their latest hypnotist.

All such programs might seem logical, and some of them might even be amusing. But they all have one thing in common: They usually don't work.

I have developed a system that does work. It's very

simple. Through much trial and error with many different systems to help patients stop smoking, I have discovered fasting to be the only satisfactory method for most people.

Plan on at least a four-day fast, during which time you will not eat or drink anything except for liberal amounts of water.

Naturally, you should check with your doctor before starting a fast. He would be wise to do a routine physical examination, a complete blood count, a routine urine examination, and an SMA-12 chemical profile to help him assess your state of general health.

If you have a serious infection, gout, diabetes, heart disease, or liver failure your doctor may not want you to fast. However, it is hard to think of any disorder that would be as potentially deadly as smoking.

Withdrawal Symptoms: During your fast you'll be so preoccupied with thoughts of food that you'll forget all about smoking, but chances are very great that you will have withdrawal symptoms while your cells make a change in their chemistry.

Most people have withdrawal symptoms which are only inconvenient: headache, insomnia, irritability, depression, weakness, queasy stomach, muscular aches, or joint pains.

A few people may have marked withdrawal symptoms, such as diarrhea, vomiting, incapacitating headaches, marked weakness, severe back pain, or confusion.

I know that doesn't sound like a very appetizing list of feel-bads, but I'm giving it to you straight. It wouldn't be fair for me to tell you your path to tobacco withdrawal is going to be strewn with dew-covered rose petals.

Don't forget, your withdrawal symptoms will be self-limiting. Knowing that the worst of the symptoms will last no more than three days should help keep up your morale and assist you in sweating through your discomforts.

It's a good idea to have a friend with you during

the fast in case your withdrawal symptoms become marked and you need assistance.

A word of cheer: The worse your withdrawal symptoms, the more important it was for you to come off tobacco.

Bufferin often helps with the less severe withdrawal symptoms: two tablets for the average adult four times a day for a day or two. Don't tell anyone I mentioned medication, because generally there are better ways of handling medical problems. (There are better ways of handling withdrawal symptoms, too, but they are too complicated for the neophyte, and I don't want to confuse you by going into them.)

You must not have even one puff of one cigarette during your withdrawal period; no cigars, no pipes, no snuff, no chewing tobacco.

Starting and Ending the Fast: As a practical matter, it's usually best to start your fast on a Thursday night. Have no more food or tobacco after bedtime Thursday night. Friday at work (your first day of withdrawal) shouldn't be too bad. Saturday and Sunday will be your worst days. If by Monday you feel quite good, you may go ahead and break your fast at that time.

Incidentally, the end of the fast is a fine time to switch over to a good diet, like the one I have outlined in Chapter 17, since the fast will have broken your allergic addictions to foods such as sugar, grains, and milk products.

Of course, you should also start on a course of vitamins and minerals, as outlined in Chapter 21. It would be well to begin vitamins and minerals at about one-quarter the given dose level and gradually build up to proper levels over a ten-day period.

Much nonsense has been written about how to end a fast—for instance, that you take only fruit and vegetable juices for the first few days. It doesn't make any difference what you end your fast with; most of my patients feel best if they have a steak. If you want to end it with a grain product like wheat, or a milk product like cheese, or a sweet like chocolate, it will give you a chance to test yourself to see whether or not you are allergic to any of these foods.

Warning: Don't test yourself for these foods while you are at work or by yourself. They may make you feel quite bad.

Your Mind Will Play Tricks: You are going to find very many good reasons for having a puff now and then. Your mind will play tricks on you. Here are some examples:

You're going to a business conference. If you do well at the conference you will get a promotion. Your income will go up 50 percent. A little voice inside tells you to have just one cigarette so you will be at your best for the conference.

Don't!

It's your birthday. This is a day to celebrate. It won't hurt to have just one.

Don't!

You've broken your ankle while skiing and it hurts like the very devil. Just one cigarette on the way to the hospital.

Don't!

Like everything else in life, you've got to choose your priorities. Once you decide what you really want, you must put that first and go after it if you are to have any hope of reaching your goal; otherwise you're only playing.

Take me, for example. I think this book I am writing is important and I want to get it done, but all sorts of things come up to distract me. I'm invited to a party given by an Arabian princess. I'm asked to give a speech in Albany. Jack Lemmon is in town appearing in a play; I might never have a chance to see him again. I get an idea for a terrific novel and think I should stop writing this book long enough to get at least the outline of the novel on paper.

We can find thousands of reasons to neglect the task at hand. But we must establish priorities; otherwise we are nothing but dilettantes pushed hither and yon by every zephyr.

I think Freud was largely a spinner of fairy tales, but he did come up with one concept I think is valid. He said that each of us has a drive toward life and a drive toward death. Something in us wants to live, but something else in us wants to die. We stand torn between these two forces.

In my view, this is a very real problem both for individuals and for groups of people. The part of you which wants to live will want you to give up tobacco. The part of you which wants to die will want you to keep smoking.

You must make an intellectual, not an emotional decision about which goal you are going to seek. Then you must force yourself to travel unswervingly toward that goal.

One important fact I must point out: Depressed people like to suffer. When you are depressed the drive toward death is greatly increased. Most people would be less depressed if they followed the diet and vitamin and mineral regime recommended in this book. Indirectly this would help them to give up smoking.

Although every cell in every person needs all vitamins and minerals, it is my impression that vitamin C is particularly helpful for people who want to stop smoking. Often taking vitamin C in doses close to 25 grams daily (divided into four doses) helps ex-smokers to stay on the wagon.

If patients have an overwhelming desire for a cigarette, taking an extra dose of 1 or 2 teaspoons (4 to 8 grams) of ascorbic acid dissolved in a glass of room-temperature water will usually banish the urge.

Smokers will be interested to know that each cigarette uses up 25 milligrams of vitamin C. If you're a three-pack-a-day smoker you'll need 1.5 grams of vitamin C daily just to stay even.

Think Cancer

We all have a psychological mechanism which helps protect us from unpleasantness. It's called denial.

When three teenagers race down a curving mountain road in three separate cars at a tire-squealing sixty miles an hour while touching bumpers, taking curves on the wrong side of the road, driving with one hand and drinking beer with the other, they know they are courting death (it appeals to their death instinct), but their mind doesn't really believe they will have an accident and die. Death is something that happens to other people, people they see on TV news programs. Death won't come to them.

You and I don't behave in such a way, because our intellect tells us that we are greatly increasing our chance of dying by driving recklessly. Still, too many people let their denial mechanism get away with telling them they won't develop cancer from smoking. Cancer is something that happens to other people.

You don't bet on the long odds when you drive—why bet on them by playing Russian roulette with cancer?

And Think How You Would Feel If . . .

Think about Nat King Cole at the pinnacle of his career, flooded with fame and money, adored by a whole nation. How did he react when he developed lung cancer? How did he feel about giving up not only his kingdom but his very life for something so trivial as cigarettes?

He must have asked himself how he could have been so stupid as to trade his birthright for a mess of pottage. He must have wept bitter tears of frustration. He had made a bargain and now there was no going back on it. He was going to die, for a cigarette!

And what about Edward R. Murrow, one of the most famous men of his times, a TV journalist who spent his time with the princes and princesses of this world and gave it all up for a cigarette?

Think about Rosemary Nay, whom you met in Chapter 1 of this book. What would she give to turn back the clock and live her life over again without cigarettes?

Are you like the teenagers who drive recklessly and court death and tell yourself it can't happen to you? Brother, it can happen to you.

The next time you light up, ask yourself if you are willing to die dead for that smoke, to have your cancer-wasted body carried away to the morgue to be shot full of embalming fluid, to have it incinerated until what was you and your life is nothing but a handful of ashes.

Tobacco is death—not a quick clean death, but a slow, expensive spirit-killing, ignoble, painful death that approaches week by week as gradually you cough up more and more blood, become unable to eat, see your strength and tissue wasting away, vomit, become blocked up or incontinent. You glance at yourself in the mirror and see the devastation.

Tobacco death is a bad death.

Vitamins and Minerals to Prevent Cancer

This is going to be a boring chapter.

How often have you turned to a new chapter and had the author tell you that you were facing dull gray?

At least I'm being honest with you. It's even going to be a dull chapter to write. I've been putting it off to the end, because I hated the prospect of wading through the references needed to give the chapter enough weight to satisfy the critics.

If you don't want to read this chapter, then read chapter 21, which will tell you how to take your vitamins and minerals. Then just take them, and believe me when I say they will in all probability help you resist cancer.

If you insist upon reading the rest of this chapter, remember that you do so at your own risk.

VITAMIN C

I can't absolutely prove to you that the big C will protect you from the other big C, but there is much clinical evidence that vitamin C not only shrinks cancerous tumors but also prolongs the life of cancer victims and may well be curative for some. I have personally seen a combination of oral and local vitamin C clear away skin cancers.

Since vitamin C is effective against cancer generally,

it is only logical that vitamin C is helpful in the prevention of cancer.

Here are a few solid points to consider.

J. W. McCormick, M.D.,[1] called attention to an important point regarding vitamin C and cancer. Cancer develops gradually from tissue that is already sick. He points out that it is the loss of collagen tissue (the hard tissue that holds the cells together), a "softening" of the tissue into "pseudo-elastic" tissue, that precedes the cancerous degeneration of the cells.

One of vitamin C's chief functions is known to be the formation of hard collagen, hard connective tissue. (This was pointed out in a different way by Ewan Cameron in Chapter 4.)

McCormick also points out that scirrhous (hard) cancer of the breast, for example, is much less malignant, much less invasive than the breast cancers which are soft.

It is very likely that vitamin C plays a strong role in the soft-hard problem, both in prevention and in treatment of cancer.

Once you begin looking through the literature, you nearly always find a few surprises. It turns out that an article by a German doctor appeared in the *Journal of the American Medical Association* (of all places!, but remember that back in 1954 vitamins were still in style and the Establishment wasn't hostile to things nutritional) on August 14, 1954, telling the results of 10 terminally ill cancer patients treated with 1 gram of vitamin C and 300,000 units of vitamin A daily. The strong feeling was that the patients improved and lived longer and that their tumors shrank. Later the number of treated patients was extended to 100, confirming the preliminary impressions.

Now, of course, we know the amount of vitamin C used was entirely inadequate.

In his book *Vitamin C, the Common Cold and Flu,*[2] Linus Pauling cites epidemiological studies showing that people who take even 100 to 200 milligrams of vitamin C daily have a lower incidence of cancer. Pauling estimates that if people would take from 1 to

10 grams of vitamin C daily they would reduce their risk of cancer by 75 percent.

Personally, I like those odds.

And remember, he's talking about odds produced by vitamin C intake alone, without any modification of the diet.

There are many papers in the medical literature that claim vitamin C helps prevent cancer.[3-12]

Viruses and Cancer

Viruses have been implicated more and more often in the production of cancer. Almost two generations ago it was discovered that the Rous sarcoma virus was involved in some animal cancers.[13]

The Epstein-Barr virus has long been known to be associated with a type of cancer found in Africa known as Burkitt's lymphoma. I know of no authority who does not accept the fact that there is an association, which is probably causal, between the herpes 2 virus and carcinoma of the cervix.

Most men working with the viral causes of cancer have heard about the French medical student who, more than a quarter of a century ago, accidentally stuck himself in the arm with a scalpel that was being used to remove a cancerous breast. He later developed cancer at the site of the injury and ultimately died as a result of the cancer.

Those who are interested in the relationship between cancer and viruses should read a recent monograph: K. Nakaraha et al., *Recent Advances in Human Tumor Virology and Immunology* (Baltimore: University Park Press, 1972).

Does Vitamin C Kill Viruses?

To answer this question in a word: yes.

One of the earliest papers on this subject was by Jungeblut[14] in 1935. He showed that vitamin C in concentrations possible in the human body kills the virus which cases infantile paralysis. There followed many other studies demonstrating the usefulness of vitamin C for treating virus infections.[15-24] Benade and others of the National Cancer Institute showed that vitamin C was very toxic to cancer cells (Ehrlich ascites carcinoma cells).[25] And so on and on into the night we could follow this subject.

Take my word for it. Vitamin C in large doses kills viruses. I know. I have seen it work.

So if vitamin C kills viruses, and keeping in mind the continued close associations found between viruses and cancer, it is certainly logical to take it as a cancer preventive.

Lymphocytes and Cancer

One of the points made by Dr. Good, President and Director of Memorial Sloan-Kettering Cancer Institute (see Chapter 14), is that lymphocytes are very important in the body's fight against cancer. I think every knowledgeable scientist involved in cancer would agree with him on this point.

During my interview with Dr. Good, he pointed out that lymph cells (these are a part of the blood cells known as white blood cells) are sometimes defective in development and unable to zero in on foreign bodies (like viruses, bacterias, and cancer cells) to destroy them—unless they have a relatively large amount of vitamin C available.

He feels that these observations (on children who were malnourished and who frequently had infections and ended up with cancer) may well mean that many people who develop cancer have defects in their lymphocytes, and that many of these defects might be correctable by the use of vitamin C.

One recent study that bears on the problem has shown that the work of the immune system (and lymphocytes are a part of that system) cannot operate properly in the guinea pig without an adequate amount of viamin C.[26]

Nitrosamines

It has long been known that nitrosamines may cause cancer. These nitrosamines form in the body when nitrates are taken with food. (Bacon and other processed meats frequently have nitrates added to keep them from spoiling.) The subject has recently been reviewed by Issenberg.[27]

It is well established vitamin C will protect animals from the carcinogenic action of these nitrosamines.[28] How many of the other 5,500 chemicals added to our food cause cancer, no one knows, since only some 800 of them have been studied to any extent. Even these studies have often been inadequate. Every year we read in newspapers about another common food additive, such as red dye No. 2, which has been taken off the market because it has been found to be cancer-producing.

Since vitamin C protects against cancer from the nitrosamines, it is reasonable to assume it also protects us against other chemical insults we unknowingly get in our "average American diet."

Bladder Cancer and Vitamin C

It is well known that the use of tobacco causes an increase in the incidence of bladder cancer in man.

I have talked with J. V. Schlegel, M.D., Professor of Urology and Chairman of the Department of Urology, Tulane University School of Medicine, about his use of vitamin C for the prevention of bladder cancer.[29] For something like ten years he has been giving his patients 1.5 grams of vitamin C daily by mouth, and he has convincing figures to prove that he is preventing cancer of the bladder with this vitamin.

VITAMIN A DEFICIENCIES

I was shocked the other day to find out that I was mildly deficient in vitamin A. I have learned many things about nutrition simply by taking different combinations of vitamins and minerals and testing myself to see what happens. I have been downing 10,000 units daily, *twice* the recommended dosage of vitamin A for many months; still, it is quite obvious that either my source is inadequate, my absorption is not what it should be, or the FDA recommendations are incorrect for me.

In a federally funded ten-state nutritional survey in 1970 it was discovered that vitamin A was one of the three nutrients most often below normal in the population.

All my new patients are tested for vitamin deficiencies. I often find vitamin A deficiencies.

Vitamin A and Carcinomas

In order to understand the role of Vitamin A in the prevention and treatment of cancer, you need to know that cancer is the general term for malignant growths that are subdivided into four different types:

Carcinoma: These are solid tumors that come from epithelial tissues: the skin, the gastrointestinal tract, the lining of the respiratory tract and the urinary system, the mucous membranes of glands, nerves, and the breasts and the genital organs. These make up about 89 percent of all cancers.

Lymphoma: These are also solid tumors; they come from lymphoid tissue, specifically from the lymph nodes and spleen. The most common forms are the lymphosarcomas and Hodgkin's disease.

Leukemia: These cancers are sometimes referred to as the "liquid" cancers, as opposed to the other forms of cancer, which are "solid." Strictly speaking, the distinction is not true, since it is not the liquid part of the blood which becomes malignant. In leukemia the lymphoid tissue and the bone marrow usually produce too many white blood cells. These immature cells are thrown into the bloodstream, hence leukemia is sometimes referred to as a form of liquid cancer. The acute, usually rapidly fatal form is seen more often in children, whereas the more slowly progressive chronic type is more common in adults. Altogether, the leukemias constitute about 4 percent of all forms of cancer.

Sarcoma: These are solid tumors that come from connective tissues like cartilage, muscle, fat, and bone. They are often very rapidly growing, hence very dangerous. Fortunately they make up only about 2 percent of human malignancies.

So What Does All That Have to Do with Vitamin A?

The point in covering the types of cancer is to show that epithelial tissue cancers (the carcinomas coming from skin, the gastrointestinal tract, the lining of the respiratory tract, et cetera) are by far the most common type of cancer (89 percent).

Vitamin A is very important in the metabolism of this type of tissue and hence is important in the prevention and treatment of all carcinomas.

On March 11, 1976, Jan van Eys, M.D., Chairman of the Department of Pediatrics at the M.D. Anderson Hospital and Tumor Institute, gave a speech in which he said: "If anyone got enough vitamin A, it would be almost impossible to have cancer of the skin and mouth." He was speaking about the protection vitamin A affords these epithelial cells. In all probability, it also protects the epithelial cells in the lungs, the gastrointestinal tract, and so on.

Mansell and his colleagues demonstrated that malignancies occurring in vitamin-A-deficient tissue grew more rapidly.[30] Cone reported fewer respiratory cancers with the use of vitamin A.[31] Rowe reported that laboratory rats on a vitamin-A-deficient diet developed malignancies.[32] Sporn and others wrote a paper stating that a vitamin A analog binds cancer-producing chemicals.[33] Shamberger stated that vitamin A destroyed premalignant cells.[34] Many reports in scientific papers state that laboratory animals exposed to cancer-producing chemicals develop cancer more often if they are deficient in vitamin A.

The list of papers on the subject could go on and on, but there's no point in citing them. I'm certain by now you're sold on vitamin A as a cancer preventive.

Just in case you're not, you should remember that Dr. Good has stated that vitamin A is very important in the production of T-cells (thymus cells), which are believed to be one of the primary kind of cells that protect us against cancer. Vitamin A also certainly helps prevent infections and probably is helpful in the prevention of kidney stones.

Finally, in closing this section on Vitamin A and cancer, let me remind you that stress, whether it be the stress of modern life or the stress of cancer, tends to deplete the body of Vitamin A.

I take this vitamin in liberal amounts, and I give it to my patients with carcinomas in massive amounts.

THE B VITAMINS

Many researchers in the field of cancer have concluded that normal cells get their energy from oxidation, whereas cancer cells get their energy from fermentation. For example, oxygen is used by the normal cells to extract energy from foods, to break foods down to carbon dioxide and water. This chemical process needs a generous supply of vitamins and minerals for it to proceed normally.

On the other hand, cancer cells get their energy from foods by a process of fermentation. They end up producing lactic acid, rather than carbon dioxide and water. The process of fermentation is a primitive form of metabolism that can proceed efficiently with smaller amounts of vitamins and minerals.

One theory is that when vitamins and minerals are lacking (as in kwashiorkor, for example) the normal cells revert to fermentation to get their energy, and thus end up cancerous. Incidentally, it is thought that hydrocarbons are carcinogenic because they damage the oxidation chemistry of cells.

This argument speaks strongly for a good supply of all vitamins and minerals for both the prevention and treatment of cancer.

An interesting paper by H. F. Kraybill, Ph.D.,[35] of the National Cancer Institute, mentions a research project in which attempts were made to induce brain tumors in laboratory animals. The researchers were unable to induce cancer unless they first put the animals on a diet deficient in riboflavin (vitamin B_2).

In some studies in which animals were given cancer-producing chemicals, those that were deficient in B_2 quickly developed cancer, but those with adequate amounts of vitamin B_2 were much slower to develop cancer.

In other vitamin-B_2-deficient animals that developed cancer, the rate of cancer growth was slowed down remarkably by the administration of vitamin B_2.[36]

It is a well-accepted fact that vitamin B_6 is very important for the proper maintenance of the immune system and that failure of the immune system is one of the important causes of cancer.

Incidentally if you increase in intake of vitamin B_6, you increase the excretion of vitamin B_2 (and vice versa), so you might possibly be running a risk of inducing cancer unless you take vitamin B_2 and vitamin B_6 in approximately equal amounts.

Choline is a vitamin important for the maintenance of healthy liver function. Cirrhosis of the liver is known to frequently precede cancer of the liver.

Even a mild deficiency of choline has been demonstrated to increase the incidence of cancer in susceptible laboratory animals. Laboratory animals with live cancer have been reported to recover with the addition of choline in their diets.[37]

Vitamin E

Much is said these days about the association between eating fats and the development of cancer (see Chapter 17), but these studies do not seem to take into account the fact that increased intake of fats increases the body's need for vitamin E, so many of the studies are worthless.

When experimental animals were given various amounts of vitamin E in their diet, it was discovered that those who received the largest amounts of the vitamin had the fewest number of cancers and their cancers grew the slowest.[38]

When chemicals that may cause cancer to develop in mice were injected into these animals after they were fed a diet heavy in fats (such as corn oil or lard), twice as many cancers developed as in those mice fed a lower-fat diet.[39] *However, the addition of liberal amounts of vitamin E to the diet of another group of mice fed a high-fat diet gave them great protection against the development of malignancies.*[40]

There are many more examples from a rich literature on the importance of vitamins in the prevention of cancer, but by now I think I have made my point: *Take your vitamins. In all probability they will reduce your chance of developing cancer.*

Minerals

In passing I would like to mention that much recent literature has demonstrated an association between the mineral selenium and cancer. In areas where there is little selenium, cancer rates tend to be high.

Generous amounts of selenium are found in brewer's yeast.

Also, many cancer patients have been found deficient in the mineral zinc, as pointed out in the interview with Dr. Good in Chapter 14. In my view most people would be best off taking zinc.

Please refer to Chapter 21 to read about the nuts-and-bolts details of taking vitamins and minerals.

So, that's about it. You can't say I didn't warn you about this dull chapter. I'm happy to say, however, that things pick up on the very next page!

21

Practical Details on Vitamin and Mineral Supplements

For Cancer Prevention

To prevent cancer, and indeed to prevent other disorders and have bloomingly good health, this is the basic vitamin-mineral supplement I give many of my patients. Most patients receiving any form of treatment for cancer would also be well advised to take these supplements. Consult your doctor to learn whether this list would be appropriate for you.

Vitamins

1. Natural vitamin A, 20,000 units daily
2. Natural vitamin D, 800 units daily
3. Hy B Complex capsule 50. Start with one daily after breakfast. If well tolerated, work up to one capsule three times a day.
4. Vitamin E, 200 units daily.
5. Very fine ascorbic acid powder. Start with ¼ teaspoon in a full glass of room-temperature water four times a day. Many people find that if they tolerate the vitamin well they feel much better if they gradually work up to 1 slightly rounded teaspoon four times a day. See Chapters 20 and 22.
6. Citrus bioflavonoid powder, ¼ teaspoon mixed in with ascorbic four times a day. If well tolerated, I go to ½ teaspoon four times daily.

7. Brewer's yeast powder, ¼ teaspoon mixed in with ascorbic acid three times daily. Gradually work up to 1 heaping teaspoon three times daily. If well tolerated, 1 heaping tablespoon three times a day is even better. If brewer's yeast is not well tolerated, I switch patients to primary yeast.

8. Desiccated liver powder, 1 teaspoon three times a day mixed in with the ascorbic acid.

9. Lecithin granules, 2 heaping tablespoons daily. I have patients eat it straight, as is, or as a cereal or sprinkled on salads or mixed in with ascorbic acid (a blender is required). Refrigerate after opening.

10. Safflower oil (cold-pressed, without a preservative added), 1 teaspoon daily, as a salad oil or on the lecithin. Refrigerate after opening.

Minerals

Mineral therapy is a bit more complicated than vitamin therapy. See Chapter 18 for advice on how to get your mineral status evaluated. It's not possible to go into the fine points of mineral supplements without first having a hair test to learn about deficiencies.

In general, I would say that avoiding processed foods (purified and manufactured foods) will do much toward giving you a good mineral intake. Yeast is an excellent source of microminerals. Desiccated liver is helpful.

Most people need and tolerate the following minerals:

1. Dolomite powder, ¼ teaspoon mixed in with ascorbic acid mixture four times daily. This is a source of calcium and magnesium and, without milk products, especially important. There is a rumor floating around that dolomite isn't well absorbed. Not true—I have tested many people before and after giving them dolomite and find the vast majority of patients absorb it very well.

2. Zinc gluconate capsule, 60 milligrams, one daily.

3. Kelp, one tablet daily. People with acne might

not do well on this because of the iodine it contains. Rarely a person will have skin blemishes from it.

VITAMINS AND MINERALS IN THE TREATMENT OF CANCER

The above-mentioned vitamins and minerals should be taken by patients suffering with cancer, with the following stipulations.

Vitamins

1. Vitamin A (natural) should be taken in large amounts, up to 200,000 units daily. *Note well:* This is a potentially toxic level. Anyone taking more than 25,000 units daily of vitamin A should be under the constant supervision of a physician sophisticated in its use.

Following are the possible side effects from large amounts of vitamin A:
A. Hair loss
B. Skin rash
C. Flaking off of skin
D. Arthritic pains
E. Enlargement of the liver
F. Swelling of the nerve head in the eyes (papilledema)
G. Retinal hemorrhages
H. Muscle paralysis
I. Double vision
J. Bulging of the eyeballs
K. Fatigue
L. Flu-like feelings
M. Abdominal discomfort
N. Severe throbbing headaches
O. Insomnia
P. Restlessness
Q. Night sweats
R. Brittle nails
S. Constipation

T. Irregular menstrual periods
U. Swelling of the ankles
V. Mouth fissures

Obviously, this is a rather formidable list. What it should say to you is that you must not take large doses of vitamin A unless you are under the direct care of a physician.

The only people who have had practical difficulties with vitamin A toxicity have been babies who were given an overdose of their vitamins, some health food faddists who consumed large amounts of the vitamin without supervision, Arctic explorers who ate polar-bear liver, and some patients of dermatologists who have continued large amounts of the vitamin without a doctor's supervision.

The rationale for using vitamin A in cancer treatment is that it increases the activity of thymus cells (T-cells) against cancer cells.

2. Vitamin C should be taken to tolerance. See Chapter 22 for details and read Chapter 23 for information about toxicity.

3. Calcium pantothenate capsules, 218 milligrams four times a day. If this dosage is well tolerated, I would double it. Some people are made tired by this vitamin. In that case, six capsules should be taken at bedtime only.

4. If I had cancer I would take an injection of 1 milligram hydroxocobalamin (a form of vitamin B_{12}) once a week. If it made me feel better I would take it as often as needed to maintain the feeling of well-being. I have one doctor's wife who must take 1 milligram twice daily by injection in order to function. I have a history professor who cannot work unless he gets 6 milligrams daily by injection.

5. I would take at least three folic acid tablets three times a day. There are those who would disagree with me about giving this vitamin to patients with cancer. Dr. Good, of Sloan-Kettering, agrees with me. We both feel cancer patients should have ideal nutrition. We also agree that we do not have the final answers. We can only make an educated guess.

Exceptions: If a patient is getting chemotherapy for leukemia, then folic acid would be contraindicated since it would defeat the chemotherapy. Should patients with leukemia who are not getting chemotherapy get folic acid? I don't know, but I would be very cautious in this area. There have been reports of leukemia patients getting worse after having received folic acid. We don't know what would happen with leukemia patients if they got folic acid while they were taking ascorbic acid for their leukemia. That is to say, we don't know whether the ascorbic acid would block any untoward effects from folic acid. No one knows the answer. Dr. Saccoman (see Chapter 7) does not give folic acid to patients with any type of cancer.

There have been reports of clusters of cancer cells being rich in folic acid, meaning they are using it for their rapid reproduction. Cancer cells steal nutrients from the healthy part of the body. Surely the body's supplies should be replenished if the body's defenses are going to work at their most efficient.

One form of chemotherapy for leukemia uses a drug which blocks the body's folic acid. Since the white blood cells desperately need this vitamin to reproduce rapidly, their reproduction is slowed down. But is the cost too great? I can only say that if I had leukemia and was not on chemotherapy, I would take the vitamins and minerals as indicated for cancer. Then I would add folic acid and check to see if it caused the white blood count to jump up. If there was a significant increase in the white blood cells after taking the folic acid, I would leave off the folic acid.

6. If I had cancer I would take an injection of 1 milliliter of crude liver extract twice a week. The reason I would use Lilly brand is because that's the brand used by Murphy (the man who got the Nobel prize for discovering that liver extracts control pernicious anemia).

Cancer patients on large amounts of vitamin C must have careful attention paid to their mineral requirements, since this vitamin tends to increase the excretion of minerals. Every patient taking this form of therapy should, in my judgment, have the hair test for minerals at the beginning of treatment and every three months thereafter (see Chapter 18).

1. Patients being treated for cancer with vitamin C should have at least ¼ teaspoon of dolomite four times a day. Many of them feel better on double this amount.

2. Most patients in this category should have zinc gluconate capsules, 60 milligrams, one capsule three times a day.

3. Other minerals must be supplied in accordance with what the hair test shows.

4. Some patients lose too much potassium during vitamin C therapy. If the patient becomes weak, he should have a serum potassium check and be given extra potassium if necessary. This is strictly a medical problem that should be handled by a physician. Patients should not take supplemental potassium without a physician's supervision. Most physicians are knowledgeable about potassium supplements.

5. I know of a doctor who uses theragran-M tablets, two tablets three times a day, for extra minerals. I find this large dose usually gives the patient nothing but a stomach ache. These tablets have a horrible brownish-red dye coating. If you decide to take them, first hold them under the faucet and work them between your fingers while running water over them to wash away the dye.

22

Albert Szent-Györgyi: On a Substance That Can Make Us Sick (If We Do Not Eat It!)

It's difficult to get Dr. Szent-Györgyi to talk about scientific subjects. I suspect he has learned that people simply don't understand what he's telling them.

I was lucky to find this article—from *Executive Health,* June 1977—in which he speaks to the general public.

I am aware that having discovered ascorbic acid did not make me into an expert on the medical use of vitamins. All the same, this work made me come in touch with vitamin C more often than I would have come without it. I had hardly announced my result when I was invited by E. Merck and Co. to come to Darmstadt, Germany, to discuss the medical uses of ascorbic acid with leading German clinicians. I did not have much to say but went all the same. I found the clinicians very nice but was shocked by their lack of biological insight and lack of interest in the basic problems. They told me that they had no need of my ascorbic acid because ascorbic acid prevented scurvy, and there was no scurvy. The logic was simple, almost irrefutable. Though I could bring up no argument against it, I felt that it was completely wrong. It was wrong because "no-scurvy" does not mean health. There is a wide gap between health and no-scurvy. Scurvy

255

is a premortal syndrome, the sign of the final collapse of the whole edifice of life. What medicine has to aim for is not "no-scurvy," but full health. I would define full health as the condition in which we feel best, work best, love best, sleep and eat best, but who knows what is "best"?

Later I learned of the other pitfalls surrounding vitamins. The whole idea of a vitamin is paradox and difficult to digest. Everybody knows that things we eat can make us sick, but it seems utterly senseless to say that something which we have not eaten could make us sick. And this is exactly what a vitamin is: *a substance which makes us sick by not eating it.*

On the Differences between Artificial Drugs and Vitamins

We usually characterize the activity of a drug by the quantity in which we have administered it to achieve a certain effect. The sensitivity of various people to our *artificial* drugs seems to be fairly uniform. Not so the sensitivity to vitamins. There seem to be people who are unable to absorb or store them, and such people may develop symptoms of a vitamin deficiency on a diet which is completely satisfactory to others. I happened to meet two such cases. The first I met thirty years ago in Belgium, where I was honorary professor and was in touch with the royal family. The Belgium cuisine is very good and the royal family had the best, and so it is likely that its food left nothing to desire. All the same, the second son of the king, the Prince of Liege, had troubles. He had temperatures, did not develop properly, and nobody knew what was wrong until the idea occurred that he might suffer from a lack of vitamin C. So he received vitamin C and in no time all his troubles were over. Later I met an almost identical case in Sweden, where the son of the Hungarian cultural attaché had similar troubles. I prescribed vitamin C and D, and the trouble disappeared.

On Flavonoids (Vitamin P)

These relations were borne out in a still more striking fashion by my studies on vitamin P. The story was this:

while I isolated vitamin C, but still had it only in impure condition, the medical clinic of my university had a patient who had strong subcutaneous capillary bleedings. Such bleedings belong to the symptoms of scurvy, so I was asked for my impure vitamin preparation, which promptly cured the bleedings. After I had isolated ascorbic acid and had it in pure form a similar patient turned up. He was given pure ascorbic acid, which was ineffective. My impure preparation was still active, so, evidently, it had to contain besides ascorbic acid some substance responsible for the therapeutic action which I had purified out of it. It was a matter of intuitive guesswork on my part to think that the active substance might have been a *flavonoid*, a member of a group of well-known dyestuffs. My *pure flavonoid* promptly cured the bleedings, as it did in other later cases. I felt very strongly that this substance had to be a vitamin, so I called it "vitamin P."

On Professional Controversies of the Past ...

There followed various professional controversies in official nutrition circles which forbade calling this substance a vitamin at all. The substance was declared useless. The situation went so far that *The New York Times* printed a front-page news article on the *"uselessness"* of flavonoids (vitamin P).

· Now, years and years later, we know that these *flavonoids* are substances which can cure or prevent cataract (see article of Roger Williams in *Executive Health*, Vol. 13, No. 3, Dec. 1976). This leaves no doubt in my mind that flavonoids are vitamins, the lack of which cause subcutaneous bleeding and cataract among other troubles.

Flavonoids are widely spread in nature and so most people take in enough of them with their food to avoid symptoms of deficiency, but those hundreds of thousands who are unable to store or assimilate the substance, or have for some other reason a greater demand, develop bleedings, cataract, and other serious troubles.

Both vitamin C and P are very cheap and have no toxic effect, unless used to great excess, so the conclusion I am inclined to draw is that one does well to make sure that one is well provided with them, even if there are no evident symptoms of a deficiency.

On the Nature of the Action of Vitamins

Another most dangerous pitfall connected with vitamins is the nature of the action of these substances. This pitfall is responsible for the fact that the real meaning and importance of vitamins is still not sufficiently recognized. This may be illustrated by the following case (concerning vitamin C) which repeats itself yearly by many thousands: Mr. X has a lack of vitamin C and contracts a cold. The cold leads to pneumonia, Mr. X dies and his body is taken to the mortuary, but it is not taken there with the diagnosis "lack of vitamin C," but with the diagnosis "Pneumonia." This does not matter for him any more, but matters for the rest of mankind, which is misled in its thinking and judgment about vitamins.

On Comparing Vitamins with Lubricants . . .

This leads me to the problem of the mechanism of action of vitamins. I could illuminate this relation by comparing vitamins with lubricants, while comparing your own body with your car. *It is wrong to look upon a vitamin as a substance which just combats specific symptoms. Like a lubricant, the vitamin makes the normal working of your body possible.* If there is not enough vitamin, the working will be disturbed, leading to all sorts of damages which may accumulate and declare themselves in an early senescence and ill health. In your car, insufficient lubrication will declare itself in the wearing out of pistons and cylinders, with the result that after 40,000 miles your car will run as if it had made 80,000, and you will look at 40 as if you were over 60.

On Being Human . . .

It is only human that we like to give thoughts to our health only after we get into trouble. Once in trouble we beg for help and are willing to do anything to get better, but we dislike to be told to do this or that to *prevent* trouble. The doctor who makes too many recommendations to prevent trouble will soon have made himself unpopular. He makes himself popular only by pulling people out of the trouble they have worked themselves into.

Our Bodies Are Much More Perfect Than We Believe . . .

After more than sixty years of intense research work in biology I am deeply convinced that our bodies are much more perfect than we believe and most of our untimely troubles are due to our abusing them. Most of this we cannot blame on circumstances. In the "have" nations, such as America, far more people die of the end results of overeating than of starvation, and a better understanding of our own body and a respect for its needs may mean a drastic reduction of self-inflicted human suffering.

On the Relation of Vitamin C to Cancer . . .

This article would have to seem very incomplete without any reference to the relation of ascorbic acid to cancer. That there is some relation has been shown beyond doubt by L. Pauling and E. Cameron (see *Executive Health,* Vol. 13, No. 4, Jan. 1977). I have worked myself on cancer for several decades, blazing my own trail. I have finished a comprehensive cancer theory which not only explains in a harmonious way the known facts about cancer but also opens a wide new way for therapy.

I regret that the technicalities involved make my theory unsuitable for the pages of *Executive Health.* I am also at a loss to say how my theory relates to Pauling's results. The mechanism of action of ascorbic acid is not sufficiently cleared up to allow correlation with my theory. My feeling is that, as I stated before, *ascorbic acid helps to keep the living machinery in good shape.* Cancer is, according to my findings, a breakdown of the normal mechanism of the cell, and so it follows that there is the less chance for a breakdown the better the condition of the whole mechanism. If we can keep the living system in good shape by providing for its needs in vitamins, then cancer will have less chance to strike. I would be inclined to explain Pauling's and Cameron's results by saying that the ordering and conserving influence of ascorbic acid may be felt even in terminal cases. It is easier to prevent than cure and so a more extensive use of ascorbic acid throughout life may lead to a considerable decrease of cancer incidence. If ascorbic acid is helpful even in a terminal case, then it may prevent cancer altogether if applied in advance, throughout life. So Pauling's and Cameron's results may have far reaching consequences.

Cancer research was hitherto greatly retarded by different factors. One factor was that, moved by the suffering this disease causes, our main concern was to cure and not to understand cancer. We forgot what Bernal told us, that *we can control only what we understand.* Cancer should be looked upon, in the first place, as a problem which has to be solved, and not merely a disease which has to be cured.

The other factor which retarded cancer research was that we asked the wrong question. We asked: why does cancer grow? Experience tells us that this is the wrong question, because surgery is based on the experience that wherever we make a cut, the cells at the side of the cut proliferate and continue to do so until the wound is healed. Then they stop. This happens wherever we cut, showing that our cells have an explosive ability to grow and multiply. The question is thus not what makes a cell grow. What makes a cancer cell grow is its innate ability to multiply. *The cancer and normal cell do not differ in their ability to grow. They differ in their ability to stop growing when no more growth is needed. The cancer cell is unable to stop. The normal cell has a brake which the cancer cell is missing.*

There are also other factors which retard cancer research and prevent new ideas from being developed. Research demands money but if one asks for a grant from any of the granting agencies one has to tell exactly what one will do and discover. Research means going out into the unknown and if one knows too well ahead what one will do and find, then it is not research at all, and is not worth doing. For this reason I was unable to get grants for the last ten years and would have had to give up research had the great American Public not come to my help most generously by supporting the National Foundation for Cancer Research, which enables me to work.

23

Detailed Instructions for the Use of Massive Amounts of Vitamin C in the Treatment of Cancer

After reading the first chapter of this book you might conclude I am a Johnny-come-lately to the world of vitamin C. Not so. I did my first research with vitamin C while still a medical student and wrote a paper on the results that was published in 1944.[1]

For more than ten years now I have been deeply involved in the practice of medical nutrition. Personally I have taken as much as 40 grams a day of vitamin C daily for long periods of time (my current amount is 26 grams a day, in divided doses), and I have given large amounts of the vitamin to hundreds of my private patients. Commonly I have prescribed 16 grams a day to patients, and often higher, up to 100 grams in some situations.

Not only have I had widespread firsthand experience with the vitamin; I have also had the opportunity to read the writings of and talk in person with those who have the widest experience with the use of massive amounts of vitamin C: Abram Hoffer, Linus Pauling, Irwin Stone, and Albert Szent-Györgyi.

Like oxygen and water, vitamin C is an indispensable part of the life of every living creature on this globe—plant as well as animal. Plants manufacture their own vitamin C with great efficiency. Animals are also able to make their own vitamin C, with three great exceptions: the fruit bat, the guinea pig, and the primates: monkeys, apes—and you and I.

It seems ironic that a goat can manufacture 13 grams of vitamin C daily (and double, even quadruple the amount under stress) and you and I are left dependent upon food for our vitamin C supply. Unwittingly, Mother Nature has dealt us a grievous blow.

How We Lost Out

Irwin Stone has estimated that sixty-five million years ago our distant ancestors, through mutation, lost the ability to form the enzyme L-gulonolactone oxidase, the liver enzyme that converts glucose into vitamin C. Why did nature play this trick on us—and then perpetuate her mistake?

We believe that our distant ancestors were living in areas with a plentiful supply of fruit. They ate so much fruit at that time that nature decided they got all the vitamin C they needed in their diets. Because there seemed to be no point in the body's manufacturing vitamin C, that ability was lost. It made no sense to carry around the hardware for providing the enzyme L-gulonolactone oxidase if it was not needed.

Unfortunately, from a biological standpoint, we no longer live in a jungle where we can walk up and pick a piece of vitamin-C-rich fruit whenever we feel hungry. Worse still, our inborn desire for sweets (put there by nature to make sure we ate fruit and took in a good supply of vitamin C) has been perverted by food processors. Now we reach for a vitamin-C-less candy bar instead of juicy vitamin-C-rich fruit.

Our biochemistry is the loser: We fail to get the massive amounts of vitamin C nature intended us to have.

But that's not the worst of it.

As I have discussed previously, when we are placed

in stressful situations—whether it be physical, psychological, radiological, or chemical—we are unable to manufacture the extra vitamin C our bodies require at that time. Everyone who has fought the battle of the fat bulge knows we tend to reach for sweets when we are under stress. It's nature's way of trying to supply us with the added vitamin C we need when stressed.

Fortunately for all of us, a clever primate by the name of Albert Szent-Györgyi discovered how to make vitamin C, so now each of us can have all we need of this remarkable substance.

Vitamin C by Mouth

Patients and physicians alike need to know a few tricks about using massive amounts of vitamin C orally.

To begin with, I must point out that anyone who simply goes to the corner drugstore and buys a supply of ordinary vitamin C tablets and starts taking 10 or more grams daily will only develop diarrhea very quickly and be forced to abandon the treatment. Powdered ascorbic acid is the best form to use.

There are three types of ascorbic acid labeled "powder." One is coarse, like sugar; another is fine, like talcum powder; and the third is very fine. Trial and error has led me to discover that, of the three, the very fine powder ascorbic acid is the best to use, because it is much better tolerated than the coarser powders. *Important*: The very fine powder should have a dull appearance; if it is shiny, avoid it.

The very fine powder might be slightly more inconvenient than the tablet or capsule, but since (unlike the tablets or capsules) it contains no binder, coloring, or lubricant, it is far better tolerated. You may have to search for the very fine powder (I know of only two sources). And I repeat: It must have a dull appearance, not shiny.

In 1970 after the publication of Linus Pauling's

book on the treatment of the common cold with ascorbic acid, there was such a demand for vitamin C that the stores in New York ran out of the very fine powder. My patients began switching to the coarse powder. At the time, I had no idea there was a physiologically different reaction to the two products. But soon my patients began complaining of all sorts of symptoms: tiredness, depression, headache, upset stomach, and others. It took me several weeks to discover why these patients, who had been making good progress, had suddenly turned sour. Finally I found the common denominator: Each had switched to the coarse ascorbic acid powder.

I took them off the coarse powder, and they immediately felt better. The very fine powder was soon available again, so they were able to start it once more.

It is only fair to say that most people who consult me are ill and that many of them have marked allergies, so it is possible the general population would not react so poorly to the coarse powder. I can speak with firsthand knowledge only about the wide experience I have had as a medical nutritionist.

While on the subject of vitamin C powder I should mention that some companies have started diluting the powder (like the heroin dealer who cuts his product) so they can make a bigger profit. One absolutely level measuring teaspoon of the very fine powder should weigh about 3.25 grams (3,250 milligrams).*

Sodium Ascorbate. Sodium ascorbate is an alkaline form of vitamin C available in very fine powder form. Again, this should appear dull, not shiny. Many patients who have had gastric or duodenal ulcers will straight ascorbic acid powder. Only trial and error will determine which form a given individual will handle best.

There is a slight difference in the weight between the very fine sodium ascorbate and the very fine

---

* With the fine (as opposed to the very fine) powder 1 level measuring teaspoon will be about 4 grams.

straight ascorbic acid powder. One absolutely level measuring teaspoon of the latter weight about 2.75 grams.

Because the sodium ascorbate is alkaline, most patients who have had gastric or duodenal ulcers will tolerate it better than the straight ascorbic acid. Some highly allergic patients tolerate the sodium ascorbate form best.

Calcium Ascorbate. Calcium ascorbate is still another form of powdered vitamin C available. When patients are unable to tolerate the straight ascorbic acid powder and cannot take the sodium ascorbate form (rarely, a person may be allergic to it; sodium is contraindicated for patients who have heart failure, high blood pressure, or some other disorder), they should be given a trial on calcium ascorbate powder.

Happily, almost everyone can take vitamin C in one form or another.

Tablets and Capsules. The tablets of vitamin C available at the corner drugstore contain binders. Chemicals must be added to the vitamin C powder to glue it together, to make it stay in one piece as a tablet. In small amounts the binder material usually does not bother people; however, when large amounts of vitamin C are taken in the form of tablets, people tend to have allergic reactions, stomach cramps, and diarrhea.

The tablets labeled "sugar and starch free" tend to be less bothersome than the regular tablets.

Many patients develop abdominal discomfort if the tablet with a brownish coating (it's usually called a "protein coating") is used.

New patients often show me capsules of vitamin C which they have been taking on their own. Some of these capsules are colored orange or yellow. True, these are pleasant to look at, but the fact is they contain dyes which can cause trouble.

If one insisted upon taking the capsule form, the clear, colorless capsule is the preferred type. Even here we may run into difficulties, however. Ingesting large amounts of the gelatin capsule may affect some people adversely.

Also, there is the problem of the dry-powder lubricant that is present in the capsules. This lubricant is added to the ascorbic acid powder to help it flow freely through the machines that pack the ascorbic acid into capsules. Some patients are allergic to the lubricant.

Time-release Capsules. Today, time-release vitamin C capsules are touted by various companies. In theory, the time-release capsules sound ideal: They are supposed to release the vitamin gradually, thus keeping a steady level in the body. This seems important in the case of vitamin C because the kidney threshold is easily exceeded and thus large amounts of the vitamin are rapidly lost in the urine.

There are several problems with the time-release capsule, however. I have already discussed the undesirability of swallowing large amounts of the gelatin that makes up the wall of the capsule. There is also a special problem with the time-release capsules: Sometimes the small pellets containing the vitamin are not dissolved by the digestive juices and pass through the body without releasing their vitamins. As you may well imagine, this is a grievous fault.

Also, one must question the theory that it is best to have a constant high level of the vitamin in the body. Research has revealed that some drugs penetrate the body cells better if the cells are hit in waves. The peaks and valleys of the body levels of the medication may thus actually aid in the drug's penetration of the cell. Whether or not this is true with vitamin C has not, to my knowledge, been demonstrated one way or the other. This is a factor to keep in mind, however.

I must admit that I do sometimes give time-release vitamin C capsules if a patient can tolerate no other form. High doses are not usually possible, however, because of abdominal cramps.

One interesting point: Sometimes a patient will not

be able to tolerate vitamin C powder in any form, but if he is given the time-release capsule (providing he can tolerate that form), he may, after a few weeks, lose his allergy to the powdered ascorbic acid and be able to take it without difficulty.

I have occasionally found another use for the time-release capsules. When a patient reaches a point in taking the powdered vitamin C where he cannot go on to a higher dose because of gastrointestinal irritation, it is often possible to give additional vitamin C by administering time-release capsules (say, six of the 500 miligram capsules) at bedtime. Dr. William J. Saccoman taught me this technique.

There are several types of time-release vitamin C. One is a clear capsule packed with colorless sand-grain-sized granules; another is a long tablet with a brown coating. Avoid the brown tablet form, the one which has what is called a "protein" coating. Most people find they have abdominal discomfort if they take large amounts of this type of vitamin C. Naturally, you will avoid any of the colored time-release capsules.

Dosages for Cancer Treatment

No one knows the best dose of vitamin C for the prevention and treatment of cancer. We know that 10 grams daily (in divided doses) will enable terminally ill cancer patients to live three times as long as the matched controls who do not receive extra amounts of vitamin C.

It is the judgment (and this hasn't been proven yet) of every physician using vitamin C to fight cancer that the more vitamin C the patient gets, the better chance he will have for winning the battle.

Dr. Saccoman, who has had considerable experience in treating cancer with massive doses of vitamin C, aims for 1 gram of vitamin C per kilogram (2.2 pounds) of body weight. Thus, a 170-pound man would take 77.3 grams of ascorbic acid daily (in divided doses).

In practice it is not usually possible to reach this figure by using oral vitamin C alone. Patients commonly develop excessive gas, nausea, or diarrhea before getting this high. Saccoman admits that this is a figure he aims for, not the figure he reaches.

Having had wide experience with the use of vitamin C for a number of disorders, I usually start patients with the straight ascorbic acid powder (it is critically important to use a very fine powder), ½ teaspoon (about 1.5 grams) in a full glass of room-temperature water four times a day (for a total of 6 grams).

If this amount is tolerated (no gas or diarrhea), then after two or three days I have the patient gradually increase the amount to 1 slightly rounded teaspoon four times a day (a total of 16 grams). Most people can handle this amount. Some patients tolerate it best by taking it an hour before meals; others do better to take it right after eating.

Often stools are slightly loose. The loose stools usually firm up after the patient has been on the ascorbic acid for six or seven days.

After reaching 16 grams daily, I usually hold the dose at that level for about a week, then start gradually going up again by adding ½ teaspoon four times daily until the patient experiences too much gastrointestinal discomfort or has excessive diarrhea, at which point I have him skip one dose and drop by ½ teaspoon four times daily.

When several weeks have passed on the tolerated dose, it is frequently possible to gradually raise it to higher levels again.

As I've already mentioned, a few people do better on the sodium ascorbate powder, especially those with a history of peptic ulcer. The sodium can be a problem for patients with high blood pressure, kidney trouble, or congestive heart failure.

An occasional patient will find a 50–50 mixture of sodium ascorbate and ascorbic acid best.

Rarely does someone tolerate calcium ascorbate best of all. Usually people are allergic to it. The reason is, I suspect, that no one has come out with a really fine calcium ascorbate powder. That which is available is shiny. The best-tolerated products are ground so fine they have a dull appearance.

My conclusions about the best-tolerated form of ascorbic acid differ from those of many of my colleagues. I think we disagree because they do not have a really good source of very fine powder.

As I mentioned, some patients, after they reach tolerance on the powder, can add two to six of the time-release (500 milligrams) capsules at bedtime. Rarely do patients tolerate this form best. After they have been on the time-release for a while they can often begin to tolerate the powder. I prefer the colorless vitamin C capsules.

At all cost avoid colored tablets and capsules of vitamin C. Avoid all tablets if possible. If you must have a tablet, be certain that it is labeled "sugar and starch free." Avoid tablets that are "protein-coated." Especially avoid powders that have fructose added to them to make them sweet.

Although I do not take care of children, those who do give the following dosage:

One gram of ascorbic acid powder per year of age (in four divided doses) up to the age of ten. For example: A six-month-old child would get about one third of a measuring teaspoon of ascorbic acid (divided into four doses) daily; a five-year-old child would get 5 grams daily (in four divided doses) of the vitamin C powder. Since there is some variation between the fine and very fine ascorbic acid (the very fine has 3.25 grams per level teaspoon, the fine 4 grams per teaspoon), it would be a good idea to get a gram scale and weigh your own. You can buy a gram scale at a head shop or at a scientific supply company. If you take your ascorbic acid powder and a measuring teaspoon to your neighborhood druggist and ask him to give you the gram weight of 1 level teaspoon of the vitamin, I'm sure he will lend a hand. Be certain, however, to weigh a sample from each new bottle of ascorbic acid you open, unless the control number on its label is the same as that on the old bottle.

When giving the vitamin C powder to a very young child, you might try putting it in his water. Later on it can be added to orange juice if the child balks at the taste of vitamin C in plain water. Sodium ascorbate powder has no taste and so it can also be given, but be sure to check with the pediatrician first, since the sodium might be a problem in some illnesses.

Be certain that children (and adults too, for that matter) have a good intake of fluids. I like adults to have at least 1½ to 2 quarts of water daily.

I can't resist adding at this point that your family dog (even though he, unlike you, can make his own ascorbic acid) will often benefit from having the tasteless sodium ascorbic acid powder mixed in with his food. Vitamin C has been found to be very helpful in preventing hip displasia in the large breeds. Massive amounts given by vein is a very good treatment for distemper . . . but that is another book!

I feel children with cancer should be pushed to tolerance when treated with vitamin C. This means that they will probably be able to take double the amounts mentioned if it is built up slowly. You must work with your child's doctor in this matter.

Citrus Bioflavonoids

In nature—and remember that everything must ultimately go back to nature—vitamin C is found closely associated with substances known as bioflavonoids.

Back in 1936 Rusznyak and Szent-Györgyi reported that the bioflavonoids (which include eriodictyol, herperidin, and rutin) did in fact have a biological function, enhancing the performance of vitamin C.[2]

Szent-Györgyi named the bioflavonoids vitamin P,

and reported that they helped decrease capillary bleeding and prolonged the life of guinea pigs that had been deprived of vitamin C for long periods of time.[3]

Z. Zloch of Charles University in Czechoslovakia demonstrated that vitamin-C-deficient guinea pigs responded better to vitamin C treatment when it was administered together with bioflavonoids rather than alone.[4] He also reported a decrease in serum cholesterol when the bioflavonoids were administered.

There is no general agreement in medical circles, however, about the usefulness of bioflavonoids. The arguments pro and con were reported in a monograph written by Shils and Goodhart.[5]

I Give Bioflavonoids with Vitamin C

Physicians who treat patients nutritionally generally speak favorably about the use of bioflavonoids *if* they have tried using them. For example, I recently attended the meeting in Palm Springs given by the Committee for World Health to celebrate the fiftieth anniversary of the discovery of vitamin C by Szent-Györgyi. At this meeting two doctors, W. D. Currier and B. F. Hart, gave talks advocating the clinical use of the bioflavonoids along with vitamin C.

In my experience, patients who improve with the addition of vitamin C to their diets (and this includes almost all patients) feel even better and have more energy if they take bioflavonoids along with the vitamin C. I have not done a controlled study nor have I performed laboratory experiments to prove my point. However, I am a very careful clinician and am my own most questioning critic.

Patients whom I see often have visited many different physicians and private clinics before consulting me. If their improvement with me were merely due to suggestion, I suspect they would have improved elsewhere.

Also, I often try these patients on a number of different diets and combinations of vitamins and minerals before I discover the correct combinations. If suggestion were healing them, they would improve no matter what I gave them. But when I double a patient's bioflavonoid or vitamin C intake (after trying a number of different changes in their vitamin regime previously) and he suddenly reports that he feels great, I know I am dealing with a biological change rather than suggestion. When I have patients leave off the added supplement, they fall back to their previous poor level of function. When the vitamin supplement is added once more and they feel improved again, I can be fairly certain that I am dealing with a biological reality.

In a TV debate a professor once argued that my good results in treating patients with nutritional supplements came only from suggestion. My reply was that for a solid week I once had patients merely come into my office, touch the hem of my garment, and leave. None of them improved.

Many times I have added bioflavonoids to a patient's regime and seen him take several steps forward in progress toward good health. I believe what I see, once I am certain I am not looking at a mirage.

The so-called pure scientists often look down their noses at clinicians such as myself and complain that our work is not scientific enough, that we do not perform enough double-blind experiments. True, we may not operate in the ivory tower of research, but that doesn't mean we are stupid or that we don't get results. They seem to forget that if we didn't make sick people well we would soon lose our following and be forced to go to work for an institution.

My Personal Experience with Bioflavonoids

For many years I had experienced a ringing in the ears, but, distracted by a busy schedule, I did not pay much attention to it. In early 1978, however, the ringing got really loud and became annoying. I began adding and subtracting foods from my diet, because symptoms like mine are often caused by food allergies. In spite of these attempts, I was unable to reduce the ringing. After ruling out food allergy, I began adding and subtracting from my vitamin-mineral regime, trying to discover if I had developed an allergy to some of my supplements or if they were somehow out of balance. I experienced no relief.

Then one morning I decided to try increasing my intake of bioflavonoids. As if by magic, the ringing had all but disappeared within ten minutes after I took half a teaspoon of bioflavonoids along with my usual dose of vitamin C. The beneficial effect has continued.

No matter how much laboratory scientists argue about whether bioflavonoids have a true effect on living tissue, my experience left me with the certain knowledge that they do have a biological effect on me.

Bioflavonoids in Cancer Treatment

There seems to be no question left about vitamin C helping cancer patients. Since many experiments have shown that bioflavonoids enhance the action of vitamin C, I think it very important that all patients, including those suffering from cancer, be given bioflavonoids along with their vitamin C.

I cannot show you a set of survival figures to prove my point, though one day they will undoubtedly be forthcoming, but since bioflavonoids are harmless, (except for allergic reactions, which are rather common) and we have good reason to think they may be helpful, they should be used.

Ewan Cameron, who has done the most work on the use of vitamin C in cancer, agrees with me that in all probability bioflavonoids would be helpful in the fight against cancer. In another fifty years there will probably be a definitive answer. Until that time, I think, common sense demands that patients suffering from cancer be given bioflavonoids along with their vitamin C.

Mr. Cameron does not use bioflavonoids, because he is interested in answering one specific question: Does cancer respond to vitamin C therapy? Giving bioflavonoids and other vitamins and minerals to his patients would cloud his research project and preclude the clear-cut answer he seeks.

How Much Bioflavonoids?

I recommend that all patients suffering from cancer take bioflavonoids along with their ascorbic acid. Only patients who are allergic to bioflavonoids should avoid them.

The preparation of my choice is the very finely powdered material labeled "Citrus Bioflavonoid Powder." (Be careful about your supplier— I understand some of it is now being diluted with lactose.) My patients are started with ¼ teaspoon dumped in the same glass used for the vitamin C. If the powder is well tolerated, I have patients increase the amount until they are getting ½ teaspoon four times daily.

Many patients who cannot tolerate the straight citrus bioflavonoid powder can successfully take a "super C-complex" capsule, which contains bioflavonoids. One to four capsules can be taken with the vitamin C powder four times a day.

In addition, just for good measure and because we might lose some of the nutrients during processing and storing, I like for patients to squeeze the juice from half a lemon into their vitamin C–bioflavonoids drink twice a day. The pulp of the lemon should be eaten, since it is especially rich in bioflavonoids. Patients usually experience a greater lift when they add the freshly squeezed lemon juice, which leads me to think they are getting extra dietary factors not present in the processed vitamin C and bioflavonoids.

If patients happen to be allergic to the bioflavonoids, they can often use the lemon alone. If they are allergic to lemon, they can sometimes use lime or sour grapefruits. (Oranges are usually not satisfactory because of their high sugar content.) Red peppers are also an excellent source of bioflavonoids, and should be used if none of the others mentioned are well tolerated.

Since allergic reactions to bioflavonoids are not rare, I want to make certain the reader understands what I mean by allergic reactions.

Most people think of them in terms of hives or headaches, or perhaps hay fever or asthma. True, these are allergic reactions, but other allergic manifestations are more common. For example, an allergic reaction to bioflavonoids (or any other substance) can simply make you feel tired or depressed or irritable.

If one of my patients doesn't feel top-notch while taking bioflavonoids (or anything else), I have him leave it off for a week, then take it again for two or three days running. By starting and stopping the substance he can discover whether he is allergic to it. If he is allergic to citrus bioflavonoid powder, he should switch to another form. Perhaps he will tolerate it well at a lower dosage, or maybe he should take it only every four or five days.

VITAMIN C BY INJECTION

Some of the technical details that follow might seem out of place in a book for the general reader, but I know from past experience that many physicians buy my books and use the knowledge gained to treat their patients. Practical points I make in my books are often not available anyplace else. Also, many patients buy my books and give them to their doctors to introduce them to the world of medical nutrition.

Medical schools do not commonly stress nutrition, and thus many physicians do not have the knowledge needed to help their patients nutritionally. However, many doctors and patients, with the help of my books, have worked together to solve medical problems by using techniques involving nutrition. Also, there are many small, but critically important, facts in this chapter that are essential for anyone using large amounts of vitamin C.

Perhaps you will recall my having mentioned in the first chapter that I started treating Mrs. Nay with intravenous sodium ascorbate. I did this because she was too nauseated at first to take large amounts of the vitamin by mouth. Many patients suffering from advanced cancer will be in a similar condition, so it is important to give the details needed for their treatment.

Let me point out that insofar as their vitamin C effect is concerned, ascorbic acid, calcium ascorbate, sodium ascorbate, magnesium ascorbate, potassium ascorbate, et cetera, are all the same. You are probably aware that ascorbic acid is merely a scientific name for one form of vitamin C; specifically, it is l-ascorbic acid (meaning levorotary). This means that under scientific tests this type of ascorbic acid rotates a light beam to the left. There is another type of ascorbic acid called d-ascorbic acid (meaning dextrorotary), which rotates a light beam to the right. The d-ascorbic acid lacks the biological effect of a vitamin. There would be no point in taking the d-ascorbic. So far as I know, it is not on the market.

Sodium Ascorbate. Sodium ascorbate is the sodium salt of ascorbic acid. As the name implies, ascorbic acid is an acid substance. When it is combined with sodium, however, it becomes slightly alkaline.

It's very easy to perform an experiment in which you change ascorbic acid into sodium ascorbate. Simply place ½ teaspoon ascorbic acid powder in a tumbler, add ½ teaspoon bicarbonate of soda, then run in some water. You will observe a fierce bubbling for a minute or two while the chemical reaction takes place. When the bubbling stops, the ascorbic acid will have become sodium ascorbate. The bubbles were made of carbon dioxide, a byproduct of the reaction.

As already noted, the sodium contained in the sodium ascorbate may pose a problem for some people. For example, if a patient has high blood pressure or is in or near heart failure, or has kidney failure, he could be made worse by giving him the sodium. So any time sodium ascorbate is administered the physician must always ask himself whether the sodium might be contraindicated.

Instructions for Intravenous Use. The sodium ascorbate form is always used when giving vitamin C by vein, because the straight ascorbic acid is too irritating.

I use a 30 milliliter single-dose vial, *without a preservative,* that contains 250 milligrams of sodium ascorbate per milliliter. *Note that it contains no preservatives.* I find that patients have fewer side reactions from the vitamin if the preservative-free type is used. However, since it contains no preservative, the entire vial must be discarded once it is opened. The physician should not use part of the vial for patient A and then save the rest to use later in the day for patient B.

Twenty cc's (5 grams) are drawn up into a 30 cc syringe using a #22-1½ needle.

In the same syringe draw up 10 cc's of preservative-free normal saline. (Sodium Chloride Inj., U.S.P., 0.9%). This solution, too, lacks a preservative, so the physician should use the entire 10 cc vial at any one time. Should any be left over, it must be thrown away.

The two products mentioned are available only by prescription.

The normal saline is added to the sodium ascorbate to dilute it so it will be less irritating to the vein. Occasionally even this mixture will cause pain in a patient with very small veins, in which case a 50 cc syringe should be used and 20 cc's of normal saline added.

For injecting in the vein, remove the #22 x 1½ needle from the syringe and replace it with a #25 x ⅝ needle. This first injection should be made slowly (taking about three minutes) to make certain the patient is not allergic to the mixture. I have observed very few allergic reactions, even though many of the patients who received it were highly allergic individuals. Some patients who were allergic to the vitamin if taken by mouth tolerated the intravenous form quite well. The only allergic reaction I have observed (and let me emphasize again that this reaction was very rare) was a slight flushing and perhaps a transient feeling of dizziness. I have all patients lie down while they get the injection.

Ideally, the injection should be given every six hours until the patient is able to take adequate amounts of the vitamin by mouth. In reality, it is usually not practical to give the injection more than twice a day. I find, however, that patients usually respond quickly and are soon able to take their ascorbic acid by mouth.

If the doctor has reason to think the patient is low in calcium, it's a good idea to give an injection of calcium* 5 milliliters in *each* hip just before administering the intravenous vitamin C.

Incidentally, this intravenous administration of vitamin C is great for treating colds, influenza, and various other viral and bacterial infections, though the vitamin should also be taken frequently and in large amounts by mouth.

I might add that I have given hundreds of intravenous injections of vitamin C without any significant difficulty. A rare patient feels better when receiving the intravenous injections in addition to the oral vitamin. I had one very allergic patient, for example, who took 30 grams daily of ascorbic acid by mouth but had a marked increase of well-being if she had a 5 gram injection once a week. Eventually the oral route sufficed.

Ascorbic acid is available in 2 milliliter ampules for intramuscular injection; however, these are not useful for the treatment of cancer, because these vials contain the straight ascorbic acid (rather than sodium

---

* The calcium solution should contain calcium glycerophosphate, 50 milligrams (in 10 milliliters); calcium lactate, 50 milligrams (in 10 milliliters); phenol, 0.25 percent; and physiological solution of sodium chloride q.s.

ascorbate). The contents of the vial should not be given intravenously.

The points made may seem small, but all of the information is of importance for physicians not sophisticated in the use of vitamin C by injection.

INTRAVENOUS DRIP

Sometimes massive amounts of vitamin C are given by vein. For example, both of the Australian doctors I talked with give 30 to 60 grams intravenously when smaller amounts of the vitamin do not control the pain of terminally ill cancer patients. They might give this amount several times a week. They seem to administer the vitamin according to what is needed to control the pain.

They have relief of pain in mind, rather than cure of cancer.

I know of only one doctor (who wishes to remain anonymous) who uses large doses of vitamin C, administered both orally and by vein, to treat cancer.* He gives as much vitamin C by mouth as the patient can tolerate and then administers 60 grams intravenously by slow drip eighty out of one hundred days.

At present I am treating Mrs. Nay with massive amounts of vitamin C by vein. Even though she is taking 48 grams a day by mouth, I am in addition giving her 60 grams a day (six days a week) by vein. I plan to keep her on this program for three months in an attempt to stop the progression of her cancer.

She will be getting about 9,000,000 milligrams (9,000 grams) of vitamin C in a three-month period!

I would have liked to place her on this program from the very beginning, but she was so tired of "doc-

---

* He is the only physician I know of who claims to cure cancer outright with vitamin C. (That is, cancers other than skin cancers. There are three doctors, of whom I am one, who have apparently cured skin cancer with a combination of vitamin C ointment and oral vitamin C.)

toring" when I first saw her that she was not interested.

Between December 13, 1977, and April, 1978, she had a slight progression of her cancer while she was on oral doses of from 36 to 48 grams a day of vitamin C.

Around July 1, 1978, she developed a chest pain (while exercising—which shows how good she felt). X ray showed more progression of the cancer and the development of fluid in her right lung.

At this point she became interested in the intensive treatment program. We started her on 60 grams of sodium ascorbate by vein six days a week in addition to the 48 grams a day she was taking by mouth.

I am happy to report that all indications are that she is responding to the treatment. She has lost her chest pain. She has now had twelve of the intravenous infusions. Another chest X ray showed the cancer has has stopped growing.

I am very impressed with the results.

Technical Details. In giving 60 grams of sodium ascorbate by vein, I used the preservative-free type mentioned earlier. This is placed in 1,000 milliliters of Ringer's lactate (a standard I.V. fluid).

First, remove the cap of a sterile bottle of 1,000 milliliters intravenous fluids. Apply Merthiolate to the top. Remove excess Merthiolate by soaking up with sterile cotton-tipped applicators. Insert a #18 gauge needle through the rubber stopper and leave it in place.

Next, using a 50 milliliter syringe and #18 gauge needle, withdraw 120 milliliters of fluid from the bottle. (If smaller-size needles are used your hands will feel as if they were beat with a truncheon by the time you finish all the mixing.)

Then place eight vials of the preservative-free solution (30-milliliter vials with 250 milligrams of sodium ascorbate per milliliter) on a tabletop. Open them and sterilize the rubber tops with Merthiolate. Remove excess Merthiolate. Then withdraw the fluid from the vial using an #18 gauge needle attached to a 50 milliliter syringe. Inject the sodium ascorbate into the bottle of I.V. fluids. Repeat until all eight vials have been added. Using sterile cotton-tipped applicators, remove any excess fluid that may have gathered on top of the bottle of I.V. fluids. Withdraw the needle that was left in place.

Apply Merthiolate once more and remove excess. Push the spike of the intravenous fluid set into the bottle. Hang the bottle on a hook located 54 inches above the patient's arm. I remove the needle that comes with the intravenous fluid set and replace it with a #22 gauge needle. At full flow with the bottle on a hook 54 inches above the patient's arm and using the #22 gauge needle, the fluid should take about two hours to go in.

I try to use one of the veins in the middle half of the arm, between the wrist and the elbow, because the patient is less likely to disturb the needle, to have it pull out or puncture the inner wall of the vein in that position.

In passing I would like to mention that massive amounts of vitamin C by mouth and by intravenous drip for about four days allows people addicted to heroin, methadone, etc., to come off the drugs very smoothly, almost without any withdrawal symptoms. Once off the drugs, they must be maintained on a good diet, adequate supplements, and 10 to 40 grams of vitamin C daily by mouth.

THIS IS IMPORTANT

Giving large amount of vitamin C tends to deplete the body of minerals, so attention must be given to mineral intake. Please read Chapters 18, 20, and 21.

If the patient does not have adequate calcium at the time of the intravenous infusion, he may go into a mild state of tetany. He will experience this as chills and muscle tremors. If this occurs, it is possible the patient could go on into convulsions, though none of the physicians using this technique has ever had such an experience with a patient.

I know of a doctor who adds 10 milliliters of a 10 percent solution of calcium gluconate into the bottle with the intravenous fluids. This will prevent tetany, but in my experience, it often gives patients an unpleasant flush and headache, and leaves them feeling weak after the treatment.

Usually I find that patients have no problem with tetany if they take ½ teaspoon dolomite powder in water four times a day. In addition, they should take 1 teaspoon of the powder just before starting the infusion.

If this does not give the patient enough calcium, give 10 milliliters of the calcium solution mentioned in footnote on p. 000 by injection in each leg beneath the fascialata (as you would a hypodermoclysis) just prior to starting the I.V. infusion.

I would suggest to any physician using the 60 grams I.V. technique that he have calcium gluconate on hand in 10 milliliter vials. Should the patient develop any signs of tetany, 5 milliliters of this material can be injected slowly into the intravenous tubing. This will promptly stop the tetany. To keep it from returning I would suggest that 10 milliliters of the other calcium solution, detailed on p. 000 be given in each leg as soon as the intravenous calcium gluconate injection is completed.

Each physician will have to learn just what type of calcium and how much needs to be given to each patient, since patients vary.

One physician, who wishes to remain anonymous, has reported that after giving the 60 grams of sodium ascorbate intravenously at frequent intervals over a period of time, he had seen a potassium deficiency develop. This has not been a problem with my patients, because I keep them off junk foods, give them a diet of meat, vegetables, fruit (all of which are good sources of potassium), and kelp and brewer's yeast, which are good sources not only of potassium but of all other minerals.

Please read Chapters 18 and 21 before employing this technique.

A Few More Small Points

It goes without saying that the patient must be in a comfortable situation. Special attention should be paid to absence of drafts and proper room temperature. Overhead lights should be turned off.

Patients must have a readily available, reliable way to signal for help if they need attention during the infusion. Someone on the physician's staff must check the patient every few minutes to make certain that all is going well, that there is no tetany beginning (it starts as restlessness), no general discomfort.

Because large amounts of ascorbic acid are dehydrating, the patient will need to drink water (through a straw) during the treatment even though getting water by vein.

The patient will probably need to pass urine once or twice during the intravenous treatment. It is most important that the patient be questioned on this point and that this need be attended to. Men can use a urinal. Some older men may have prostatic hypertrophy and will need to sit on the side of the bed or even stand up to void. Women should be assisted to their feet and then a bedpan should be placed in a nearby chair for them to use.

Two people are required to help patients void. One should hold the arm into which the fluid is flowing to make certain the needle is not stressed in such a way that it will pull out of or be pushed through the vein.

It is usually perfectly safe for patients to go home alone. At first, however, until this is established, someone should call for the patient to assist him home.

Vitamin C Ointment

I have been told of a doctor, who wishes to remain anonymous, who has apparently used vitamin C ointment to treat the skin cancers of between 100 and 200 patients, and has had excellent results, even with advanced cases. I discussed this form of therapy with Dr. Archie Kalokerinos of Sydney, Australia, who has treated a number of skin cancers with a vitamin C ointment. He too reports excellent results.

I have personally treated 3 patients with skin cancer by using vitamin C ointment, and I too have been very pleased with the outcome. All of the cancers completely disappeared.

I used an ointment made up of 30 percent (by weight) very fine ascorbic acid powder in a water-soluble base (Unibase). This should be made up fresh by the pharmacist and kept in the refrigerator. The ointment is gently rubbed into the skin cancer six to eight times daily. If the 30 percent ointment proves irritating, then a weaker one (all the way down to 10 percent) can be used, although I have had no personal experience with the weaker type.

It is possible that some patients will tolerate a sodium ascorbate ointment better than a straight ascorbic acid ointment. Theoretically, it should work just as well, although this is only speculation on my part, since I have had no firsthand experience with it.

24

Are Large Amounts
of Vitamin C Toxic?

Many familiar things are toxic.

You've been around air for a long time, but did you know that air in improper amounts can be toxic? For example, that if you breathe rapidly in and out for a short time you will feel dizzy? Some people will pass out if they continue. Can't you see the headlines:

SCIENTISTS DISCOVER BREATHING CAN BE
HARMFUL TO YOUR HEALTH!

If you read such a headline you might glance through the article, but you wouldn't be terribly alarmed, because you have had a great deal of personal experience with breathing air and you know what air will do and what it won't do. You don't have to depend upon research to tell you about the effects of air on your body.

We could talk about the toxicity of sugar—how it makes you fat and how the excess weight often leads to diabetes, high blood pressure, heart attacks, and strokes.

And most people are aware that common table salt is very toxic for people with certain types of heart disease and those suffering from high blood pressure.

And water—did you know that you can die from excessive intake of water? I'm not talking about the cup of water that may kill you if you inhale it, but rather the drowning that can come from excessive dilution of your body chemistry if you drink too much water.

And carrot juice—did you know that a death has been reported from drinking too much carrot juice?

And alcohol—if you can get your worst enemy to drink two quarts of bourbon you can very likely do him in once and for all. If you want to be more subtle about it, give him modest amounts of alcohol over a long period of time and let him die from cirrhosis of the liver.

Compared to the toxicity of air, sugar, salt, water, carrot juice, and alcohol, vitamin C is child's play. There is a report of a patient who tried to commit suicide by O.D.ing on vitamin C. He took something like 150 grams (about 38 teaspoons). All he got was nausea and the trots.

THE ELEVEN TRUE TOXIC EFFECTS FROM MASSIVE AMOUNTS OF VITAMIN C

There are eleven legitimate toxic effects from massive amounts of vitamin C. Those of us who have been practicing medicine for many years and have used vitamin C in massive amounts for our patients all agree that there are only eleven toxic effects. Abram Hoffer, a Canadian physician, has used vitamin C in mega amounts for his patients since 1950. He thoroughly agrees with the above statement.

The true toxic effects are:
1. Excessive gas
2. Nausea
3. Diarrhea
4. Urinary burning and frequency (rare)
5. Rarely, vitamin C in large amounts may irritate the mouth
6. Ascorbic acid may irritate a gastric or duodenal ulcer. I have also had patients with inflammation of the esophagus who were unable to take ascorbic acid.

7. Dentists sometimes express the fear that ascorbic acid may injure the tooth enamel.

8. Dehydration

9. Loss of minerals

10. Temporary initial increase in pain in a few patients with terminal cancer

11. Hemorrhage, in advanced cancer patients only. (See the discussion that follows.)

The first four side effects are never serious or in any way life-threatening, and can usually be got around by temporarily reducing the dosage of vitamin C or switching to a different form.

I have seen vitamin C irritate the mouth only once or twice, and it was never a serious problem. When this happened the patients were not properly diluting the vitamin C. It should be taken in a full glass of room-temperature water. If more than 30 grams a day is taken it is sometimes a good idea to divide the daily dose by eight rather than four. (A glass straw may also be used.)

If vitamin C irritates a gastric or duodenal ulcer, this can be circumvented in one of several ways. The alkaline form of vitamin C can be used: either sodium ascorbate or calcium ascorbate (see Chapter 21). A time-release form may also be useful. Some of my patients with ulcers take the acid form of vitamin C without any difficulty.

I have never seen vitamin C damage tooth enamel, but dentists sometimes worry about this. The solution is simple: Take the vitamin through a straw or else rinse the mouth with water containing bicarbonate of soda (common baking soda, *not* baking powder).

Dehydration is not a large problem. The obvious solution is to have the patient drink more water. The average person will be thirsty when taking large amounts of vitamin C and automatically will take more fluids. For patients who tend to retain water in their bodies (menstruating women, certain patients with allergic edema, some types of heart disease) this diuretic effect of vitamin C may actually be an advantage.

Old people or desperately sick patients who might be confused and out of touch with their bodily signals should be given special attention. Their daily water intake should be measured and recorded. Generally they should have two quarts or more a day. Any intravenous fluids they get with their vitamin C should not count toward this goal.

Dehydration may be a problem with patients who are getting large amounts of the vitamin by vein unless they drink liberal amounts of water while they are getting their intravenous drip. If they are allowed to become dehydrated at this time they will feel weak. Make certain they drink water while receiving the infusion.

With large doses of ascorbic acid, especially when given both by mouth and by vein over a long period of time, patients do tend to lose body minerals. This is one compelling reason why these patients should be kept off junk foods. In my somewhat strict view, junk foods include everything except fresh meat, fresh vegetables, fresh fruits, and chlorine-free, fluoride-free water. Junk foods have usually been stripped of many of their minerals.

We think of milk as being the only common source of minerals in our diet. Not so. Did you ever stop to think where the cow gets the minerals she needs to make the milk? Certainly not from pizza.

Dolomite, brewer's yeast, primary yeast, torula yeast, and kelp are all excellent sources of minerals (including the microminerals). In addition, almost everyone in our society would do well to take about 60 milligrams of zinc gluconate daily. Most patients with cancer should have triple this amount. Of course, fresh vegetables and fresh fruits are a source of minerals.

As I pointed out earlier, I feel everyone should have a hair test for minerals. Specific deficiencies should be attended to based on this laboratory evidence.

If a patient gets to feeling better on large amounts of vitamin C and then, after a period of time, begins to complain of fatigue, he should be considered to be suffering from mineral deficiencies until proven otherwise.

Cancer patients receiving long-term intravenous vitamin C will usually do much better if they get ¼ to ½ teaspoon dolomite in water four times daily and 1 teaspoon just before starting the drip. If possible, they should also take one kelp tablet three times daily, as well as powdered yeast.

I know of one doctor who gives patients two theragran-M tablets three times a day as an additional source of vitamins and minerals. However, I have found this upsets many patients.

Once in a while a patient may need an injection of calcium to prevent tetany (a form of muscle spasm) while getting intravenous vitamin C in amounts of 30 grams or more.

If potassium is needed above the amounts mentioned in the supplements discussed, this is strictly a medical problem that should be addressed only by a physician.

Cameron reports that some of his patients with widespread cancer feel a very temporary increase in pain when first placed on his vitamin C regime. This disappears within several days. It is simply a period that must be got past.

By far the most serious complication from massive amounts of vitamin C is hemorrhage. Apparently it is not a rare occurrence among patients with far-advanced cancer. Both Kalokerinos and Cameron report this serious complication.

In regard to hemorrhage, let me stress two points.

First, the hemorrhages have occurred only in terminally ill patients with widespread cancer throughout their bodies.

Second, the hemorrhages have been reported to be due to shrinkage of the cancerous growth. If cancer happens to be wrapped around a blood vessel and the cancer shrinks, it may pull on the blood vessel and cause it to rupture.

It hardly seems fair to fault vitamin C for shrinking cancerous tumors. If anything, this is good proof that it is effective against cancer. In my view this is an acceptable risk that simply must be assumed.

There may be, however, two ways to reduce this risk. Szent-Györgyi and many others have reported that vitamin C alone will sometimes not prevent the symptoms of scurvy, including the hemorrhages which may occur. The addition of bioflavonoids to the vitamin C has resulted in cessation of these hemorrhages, however. Therefore, as I've said, I make it a point to give bioflavonoids to all patients on vitamin C. Most of them start on ¼ teaspoon citrus bioflavonoid powder in water four times a day. If this is well tolerated I have them increase the dosage to ½ teaspoon four times daily. Those doctors reporting the hemorrhages in patients with advanced cancer have not been using bioflavonoids.

One other possibility for reducing the likelihood of hemorrhage is to start the terminally ill cancer patient off on relatively small amounts of vitamin C (say, 1 gram four times a day) and gradually, over a week or two, build up to the therapeutic range. This method has not been tried yet, but I think this is a reasonable recommendation. In the future I expect to follow this plan when dealing with terminally ill patients who have widespread cancer.

You will note in the Appendices of this book that Cameron reports quite a number of terminally ill cancer patients got relief from pain. Also, quite a number of his patients did not get relief. I think the problem is that he did not use a high enough dose of the vitamin. Others (who are using from 30 to 60 grams by intravenous infusion plus all the patients can tolerate by mouth) tell me that the pain relief has been almost universally dramatic.

The last thing one must bear in mind is that advanced cancer represents a desperate situation in which almost any risk of therapy is acceptable. If something is not done, all of the patients are going to die.

If a patient places his last bet on ascorbic acid (because there are no other bets open) and loses, then we must somehow be philosophical about it. However crass it may sound, death by hemorrhage is not a bad way to die compared to some of the other ways patients die from advanced cancer.

CAUTIONS IN THE USE OF LARGE AMOUNTS OF VITAMIN C

Again, let me advise you to read Chapter 23 in which I discuss in detail the uses of large amounts of vitamin C.

Large Doses of Vitamin C May Produce Pentosuria

This is a harmless form of sugar in the urine, but if a person happens to be a diabetic and is testing his urine with a glucose oxidase method to judge how much insulin to take, the tests may give false positives. Check with your doctor on this point.

Interaction with Warfarin

Coumadin is one trade name for warfarin. The popular term for this anticoagulant is "blood thinner." It's given to some patients who have a tendency for their blood to clot abnormally, especially if they have had repeated thromboses or have had a coronary heart attack. Check with your doctor carefully and be certain he takes prothrombin tests frequently if you are on warfarin and start taking large amounts of vitamin C. (The same holds true for niacin, one form of vitamin B_3.)

Rebound Effect

You will read about this effect in the paper by Stone and Hoffer at the end of this chapter. Just to make certain you have the problem clearly in mind, let me clarify what is meant by rebound effect.

If large amounts of a substance are taken over a long period of time, the body chemistry adjusts to make use of this generous supply. If, on the other hand, the substance is present only in small amounts, the body makes do by utilizing alternative chemical processes.

For example, if you eat a diet high in carbohydrate and then suddenly switch to a diet low in carbohydrate (high in proteins and fats), it takes your body a few weeks to make the transition.

Here's a more specific example: If bacteria are grown in a medium rich in sucrose (table sugar) and then suddenly changed to a medium rich in fructose (fruit sugar), they will need time to adjust to the new diet.

While on the sucrose diet the bacteria's enzyme systems for handling the fructose will be greatly reduced in number. When the bacteria are switched to a rich fructose diet, they must manufacture more fructose-functioning enzymes before they can handle the new diet efficiently.

Gradually, as the bacteria continue on the new diet, the fructose-handling enzymes will increase in number and the sucrose-handling enzymes will greatly shrink in number.

Scientific papers have suggested that people suddenly taken off large amounts of vitamin C may suffer from vitamin C deficiency. This problem is especially interesting in regard to the newborn baby. What if the fetus is being carried by someone who takes large amounts of vitamin C and then the baby is born and placed on a bottle? The new food will contain very small amounts (possibly none at all) of vitamin C. Will the sudden reduction in vitamin C intake harm the baby?

There have been conflicting reports in the scientific literature on this point.[1]

What to do?

I haven't given patients large amounts of vitamin C, measured their vitamin C serum and white blood cell levels, then taken them off vitamin C and repeated the studies, so I cannot answer the question from firsthand experience.

I have had patients on large amounts of vitamin C who suddenly stopped taking it, for one reason or another. None of them suffered any ill effects so far as I could tell.

I do think it makes biochemical common sense, however, to come off high doses of vitamin C slowly if you are going to stop it. Since it's important to change other dietary factors slowly, why shouldn't it be important in the case of vitamin C? It's easy enough for most people to gradually reduce their dosage of vitamin C over a period of several weeks if they choose to come off it.

The newborn baby has a special problem, however, since he is forcefully and almost totally withdrawn at a critical time in his life, when he goes from the easy life of the womb into the harsh realities of the cold outside world.

I would advise pregnant women to take their ascorbic acid and then, when the baby is born, start giving it to him. A newborn can easily take 0.5 gram of ascorbic acid daily. That's ¼ teaspoon. It should, however, be divided into four doses: $\frac{1}{16}$ teaspoon four times a day. It can be put in his water. Chances are he will accept it if it's well diluted. If he finds the taste unacceptable, he can be given the tasteless sodium ascorbate, so long as there is no reason for him to avoid the sodium. Calcium ascorbate can also be used as an alternative. *Please consult your family doctor or pediatrician on these (as well as all other) points.*

Reported Toxic Effects Found False

Although all of the following toxic effects of vitamin C have been reported in the news media, all of them have turned out to be false. Here's the list: destruction of vitamin B_{12}, kidney stones, abortion, precipitation of attacks of gout, and cancer.

That's quite a list.

You may be quite certain that if these reports were true the FDA would have banned the sale of ascorbic acid long ago, because the federal government, while it supports the tobacco and sugar cane grower, is very hostile toward all aspects of nutrition that are not academically oriented.

Now let's take up the false side effects one at a time.

Vitamin C Destroys Vitamin B$_{12}$

The suggestion that vitamin C destroyed vitamin B$_{12}$ was reported more than twenty years ago.[2]

Investigators who repeated the studies, using improved laboratory methods, reported no significant destruction of vitamin B$_{12}$ by vitamin C.[3]

Large Doses of Vitamin C Cause Kidney Stones

Soon after Pauling's book on the use of vitamin C for the treatment of the common cold appeared, a host of editorial comments appeared in medical journals warning about the possibility that large doses of vitamin C might cause kidney stones. This speculation came about because it is well known that a large intake of vitamin C causes patients to excrete increased amounts of calcium oxalate, cystine, and uric acid, each of which can be a compound found in kidney stones.

The authors of these attacks were all men who lacked wide experience in its use. They were giving an armchair opinion, so to speak. As everyone with any street smarts knows, there's a world of difference between what is theoretically true and what is true in reality.

The truth is vitamin C does not increase the incidence of kidney stones. How do I know? I've given vitamin C to hundreds—no, thousands of patients in large doses over the past twelve years. I have had only one patient develop a kidney stone during this period. That patient had a small stone, passed it without much difficulty, and, so far as I know, has never had any more trouble with kidney stones. After passing the stone she kept right on taking vitamin C, with my blessing and the blessing of her urologist.

Considering the number of patients I see in my large practice, one would guess that chance alone would have sent more than one kidney stone my way during the last twelve years. I think that far from causing kidney stones, the large amounts of vitamin C my patients take protect them from kidney stones.

How?

First, ascorbic acid acidifies the urine. It is well known in the medical profession that patients have fewer urinary infections when the urine is acid. Indeed, mandelic acid is a standard prescription frequently given patients with urinary infections.

Second, ascorbic acid (as well as other forms of vitamin C) is antibacterial in itself.

Third, patients who receive adequate amounts of vitamins, including generous amounts of vitamin C, have better resistance against infections. Their immunological response is better. The efficiency of the white blood cells is increased. Both are crucially important in the body's fight against infection.

Why all this about infection when we were talking about kidney stones?

The reason is quite simple: Most urologists agree that a low-grade kidney infection is an important cause of kidney stone formation. The infection seems to be the irritation around which the stones form, just as an oyster makes a pearl only when a grain of sand or some other such irritant is present.

Another point: Vitamin C in large doses has a diuretic effect. That is, it tends to flush water out of the body through the kidneys. This extra water through the kidneys tends to keep them free of stone formation. Every patient who has been bothered by kidney stones has been advised by his urologist to drink more water to aid in this flushing process.

Sometimes a new patient with a known kidney stone

consults me. I try giving him sodium ascorbate (an alkaline form of vitamin C) if he has a history of uric acid or cystine stones, because these stones are thought to form less easily in alkaline urine. Sometimes I find that the sodium ascorbate will not keep the urine free of infection. In these cases, I go back to ascorbic acid even if the stone formation is due to uric acid or cystine.

Abram Hoffer has used ascorbic acid in massive amounts in thousands of patients over the past twenty-nine years and tells me his clinical experience is similar to mine; if anything, he has seen far less stone formation in his patients than he would expect from statistical chance alone. Like me, he thinks the idea that high doses of ascorbic acid cause kidney stones is nonsense.

A physician—who wishes to remain anonymous—with widespread experience in the use of massive amounts of vitamin C for more than thirty years, feels that, if anything, vitamin C retards kidney stone formation.

During the past five years, a growing number of psychiatrists have begun to use megavitamin therapy for emotional illnesses. Included in their regime are large doses of vitamin C. Their patients have not been bothered by kidney stones.

Lewin, in his excellent book on vitamin C, states that calcium oxalate is more soluble in the type of acid urine created by ascorbic acid and thus calcium oxalate stones are less likely to form when the vitamin is taken.[4]

You can bet that if the antivitamin establishment could find any proof that vitamin C causes an increase in the incident of kidney stones they would be flooding the media with that information and the FDA would be making vigorous efforts to take the product off the market.

The truth is that vitamin C in large amounts does not cause kidney stones. In all probability, taking vitamin C in large doses protects against kidney stones.

I take vitamin C in large amounts. If I had any idea whatsoever that it was going to give me kidney stones, you can bet I would carefully avoid it.

Large Doses of Vitamin C Cause Abortions

This untrue "fact," often dwelled upon by the anti-vitamin establishment in their newspaper columns, got started in 1966 with the publication of a paper in the Soviet Union reporting the work of Samborskaya and Ferdman,[5] who stated that 20 women, aged twenty to forty, were given 6 grams of vitamin C daily for three days after their menstrual periods had been delayed ten to fifteen days. Sixteen of them menstruated after having received the ascorbic acid.

You don't need to be a biostatistician to spot the holes in this paper. They didn't even do pregnancy tests on the women. Linus Pauling wrote to the authors to clarify this point. All he got in reply was another copy of the paper!

We know that women having irregular menstrual periods often revert to normally spaced periods after getting proper nutrition, including vitamin C. I suspect that these women were simply deficient in vitamin C and began having normal periods after receiving the vitamin.

In 1970, Lahann reviewed the medical literature in regard to vitamin C and menstruation. He discovered many medical reports of improved menstruation after administration of 200 to 1,000 milligrams of vitamin C daily.

But the best proof of all that vitamin C does not cause abortion lies in the clinical experience of those of us who have been giving large daily amounts of vitamin C to many thousands of women. We simply haven't seen an increase in the incidence of abortion in these women. We don't need to read the literature to learn the answer. We know it because we've seen for ourselves.

Large Amounts of Vitamin C Cause Gout

Again, those of us who have been using vitamin C in large amounts in many patients over a period of years simply have not had our patients developing gout.

One of my patients came to me with a uric acid blood level of 19 milligrams per 100 cc (normal levels are 2.5 to 8.5 mg%). This is an astronomically high level, the highest I remember seeing. With massive amounts of vitamin C this level fell to normal in a few months.

Just last month I saw a patient with a uric acid level of 8.6 mg%. He too was given large amounts of vitamin C. When I tested him a month later, his level had fallen to 7.5 mg%. (Incidentally, his serum cholesterol had fallen from 258 mg% to 217 mg% in spite of a diet consisting mainly of animal fats and animal proteins!)

Large Doses of Vitamin C Cause Cancer

I think the best answer to this myth comes in a paper published by Irwin Stone and Abram Hoffer in the *Journal of Orthomolecular Psychiatry,* volume 5, no. 3 (1976), which follows.

The Genesis of Medical Myths

A medical myth is an aggressive defensive device used by orthodox medicine to retain the status quo and impede progress in the introduction of new and valuable therapies. It is the same technique and disorganized thinking as that used by the surgeons of a century ago in savagely refusing to wash their hands before performing surgery.

The myth originates in some inadequate sloppy in vitro or animal experimental work from which unwarranted broad conclusions are drawn as to possible effects on man. There is never any hard human evidence involved, just pure speculation. The second step is that the news media pick it up and, being more interested in sensationalism than in facts, magnify these speculations and terrify a gullible public. Further repetition of these unwarranted conclusions by the medical press gives them the status of medical dogma to be quoted and requoted.

Megascorbic and megavitamin preventive medicine and therapy has been particularly subjected to this sort of attack in the past. Three more biased reports have recently appeared which will form the basis of future attacks. They suggest that "massive" doses of ascorbic acid will cause cancer, will cause gout, and will cause scurvy in infants of mothers consuming these doses. These speculations will surely be accepted, not as ideas, but as facts, and the public will be solemnly warned to avoid these high dangerous doses. This, in spite of 23 years of clinical observations (AH) on several thousand patients consuming "massive" daily doses of ascorbate, which have failed to reveal a single case of scurvy in infants or any serious toxicity because of this ascorbate intake (Hoffer, 1971). For this reason it is essential to examine closely the three reports.

The publication in the April 22, 1976, issue of *Nature*, by Stich et al. (1976) of the paper, "Mutagenic Action of Ascorbic Acid," has started a new wave of unwarranted criticism and sly innuendo against the use of "mega" doses of ascorbate in humans. Even the title of their paper is biased and misleading, because they promptly show that ascorbic acid is harmless and *not* mutagenic and only becomes so when it is chemically oxidized or mixed with soluble copper ions, "in vitro." The responsibility for this unconscionable laxity in title must be shared both by the authors and the editors of *Nature*.

It has been known for many years that the oxidation products of ascorbate are toxic to humans. In fact, the main reason that the several oxidation-reduction (O-R) systems were evolved during the early evolution of life on this planet (Stone, 1972) was to maintain the O-R potential of the protoplasm at the optimal low levels and protect it from oxygen toxicity. This protection was so important that many biochemical systems were evolved for this purpose. They include, besides the ascorbate-dehydoroascorbate system, back-up systems like the sulfhy-

dryldisulfide, the cytochromes, the reduced polyphenoloxi-
dized polyphenols and other sulfhydryl-containing proteins
rich in cysteine. One-and-a-half grams per Kg of dehydro-
ascorbic acid—the oxidized form—will produce diabetes
in rats. This is prevented by the presence of reducing compounds such as the sulfhydryls.

Stich et al. found:

1. Ascorbic acid alone and "not oxidized" did not have
any mutagenic effect.

2. Cultured human fibroblasts treated with oxidized
ascorbate or with a mixture of ascorbic acid plus the oxidation catalyst cupric sulfate for two hours increased DNA
fragmentation and increased repair synthesis and chromo-
some aberrations. Cupric sulfate alone had no effect.
Flushing nitrogen through the ascorbic acid solution neu-
tralized the effect. The amount of oxidized ascorbic acid
required is high compared to the amount of a known
mutagen.

These findings prompted these authors to conclude "the
potential mutagenic capacity of ascorbic acid products
should be taken into consideration when a potential health
hazard, due to the addition of relatively large quantities
of vitamin C to food products which contain nitrosamine
compounds, is evaluated."

But they also caution, "It is difficult to evaluate the
degree of genetic hazard posed by vitamin C, its decom-
position products and its interaction with metal ions in
man.

"A too simple application of these in vitro data to man
can lead to erroneous conclusions. Catalyses may inhibit
ascorbic–initiated DNA cleavage within the human body.
Metabolic products of ascorbic acid may reach the intra-
nuclear DNA molecules only, if present in excessive
amounts. The ascorbic acid–metal mixtures may have no
effect because of the lack of free cupric or ferric ions
within the cells."

As is often the case, a finding made from pure cells in
pure culture which indicates a *possibility* of a deleterious
effect is immediately translated by many as an event which
will occur with a high degree of probability. This pre-

liminary report which still must be checked by other laboratories will be jumped upon with enthusiasm by those who erroneously believe that doses of ascorbic acid are useless therapeutically, therefore it is fair game to use every possible shred of evidence, no matter how slender, to damn these high doses.

This has already happened, and in a few days we have received worried letters from correspondents, physicians, and patients. For example, it was reported in the *New York Times* that Dr. R. San, not a clinician, suggests that people should avoid massive doses of vitamin C. But he does not define what a massive dose is. Also in the Swedish paper "Sydsvenska Dagbladet" for May 21, 1976, the headline is "Too much C-Vitamin can cause cancer." Under the lead it says, "If you eat too much of the C Vitamin you will run a risk for cancer. This is claimed by a team of Canadian researchers." There was a second headline, "Do not prevent colds with C-Vitamin." "It can be dangerous to eat too much of the C-Vitamin. It can cause fetal cancer and fetal malformation." The June 17, 1976, *New York Times* carried an article headlined, "Researchers find large doses of Vitamin C may damage gene material." *The N.Y. Times News Service* distributed this article, so it also appeared in many smaller local papers.

These are samples of how a simple finding is finally presented to the public. The newspaper conclusions are, of course, nonsensical.

It is clear that ascorbic acid alone (free of oxygen and free of ionized copper) is nontoxic. It is equally clear that ascorbic acid is readily oxidized by oxygen when catalyzed by cupric ions. This is why flushing out the solution with nitrogen prevented any effect. We can then conclude that, not ascorbic acid, but some of its oxidation products are weak mutagens.

Because of a 60-million-year-old genetic defect, humans have been reprived of the ability of making their own ascorbate in their livers. The other mammals for the past 165 million years have been making it in large daily multigram levels, in the daily range that Stich et al. and others consider "dangerous." Ever since humans and their hominid ancestors have been on this earth they have suffered constantly and severely from this genetic defect that pre-

302

vented them from adequately protecting themselves against this oxygen toxicity and other forms of stress. One of the main reasons for supplying these large daily doses of ascorbate to humans is to correct this genetic disability and keep the ratio of oxidized products of ascorbate at a minimum by having an adequate large excess of the reduced form of ascorbate always present. In case anyone has forgotten their elementary facts of physical chemistry, it is the ratio of the components of an O-R system that determines the O-R potential, and healthy human tissues demand a high ratio of reduced ascorbate and a low ratio of the oxidized forms.

Stitch et al. in their research protocol flew in the face of these facts and rigged their experimental conditions to make sure the ascorbate was thoroughly oxidized. Their few "in vitro" tests showed that the reduced ascorbate was virtually non-mutagenic, while their oxidized forms showed the effect they were looking for. This is something that the physiology of the mammals has known for the past 165 million years.

The mammals found this out 165 million years ago and have been producing ever since the high levels of ascorbate that the doctors consider "dangerous." When the mammals appeared they had to make more ascorbate to survive. They did this by changing the site of synthesis of ascorbate from the small kidneys to the liver, the largest organ in the body (Stone, 1972), and also developed a new physiological feedback mechanism to produce more ascorbate under stress (Subramanian et al., 1973). Any mammal that couldn't do this didn't survive and became extinct. Can anyone argue with the results of this "in vivo" test that has been going on for 165 million years?

While we are on the subject of evolution, humans also evolved another protective mechanism against oxygen toxicity by conserving and reusing the bare subsistence levels of ascorbates that are normally found in their bodies as a result of their genetic defect. A human enzyme utilizing sulfhydryl cofactors is present which converts oxidized ascorbate back into the reduced form as long as sulfhydryl compounds are available. This, of course, was not part of Stich et al.'s experimental "in vitro" protocol.

The summary of the paper, "Association between drugs

303

administered during pregnancy and congenital abnormalities of the fetus," Mathilda M. Nelson, John O. Forfar (1971) contains the statement, "On the other hand, deficiencies such as those of ascorbic acid and folic acid may have a teratogenic effect." Another "in vivo" bit of evidence in favor of ascorbate.

While Stich et al. suggested caution in applying their "in vitro" test results on tissue cultures and typhoid bacteria to "in vivo" conclusions in humans, such warnings are never heeded by the press. They are more interested in sensationalism at the expense of facts. The damage has already been done in the public mind with the newspaper articles stating that large doses of ascorbate increase the risk of both defects and cancer, when just the opposite is the truth. The 1971 paper showed that birth defects increase from a deficiency of ascorbate, and recent work on cancer shows that large doses of ascorbate are being used to prevent and treat cancer successfully (see article on cancer by Stone, this issue).

The choice of test material in Stich et al.'s Table 2 (salmonella typhimurium) was poor because of ascorbate's known toxicity for typhoid-type bacteria and the many references where ascorbate has been used therapeutically in typhoid fever (Stone, 1972a).

From the in vitro findings, which still must be validated, there is a mega leap to conclude that dosages commonly used will cause cancer in man. There has been no report anywhere in the literature that this has occurred. There is little doubt that if there were even a single case, it would have been reported in the medical literature and widely disseminated in the press. On the contrary there are a number of reports that ascorbic acid has anticarcinogenic properties. Who is one to believe—a tentative suggestion based upon a study of cells "in vitro" which still requires a lot of investigation, or the vast cumulative experience of thousands of physicians on millions of people among whom not a single case of cancer attributable to ascorbic acid has been found? Also clinical evidence is accumulating that large doses of ascorbate can prevent cancer and is used in cancer therapy.

In a second similar type of paper, Stein et al. (1976) summarized the results of their research as follows: "Two to six hours after the ingestion of 4.0 g of ascorbic acid, the fractional clearance of uric acid increased to 20.2%–21% of the control value." "Ascorbic acid did not diminish proteinbound uric acid. In 3 subjects who ingested 8.0 g of ascorbic acid for 3 to 7 days the serum uric acid decreased by 1.2 mg to 3.1 mg/dl as a result of sustained uricosuria." "Theoretically it could precipitate attacks of gouty arthritis or renal calculi in predisposed persons."

Ascorbic acid is relatively nontoxic. In this way it does not resemble any of the drugs normally not found in the body. In order to establish it as a drug, since physicians are unused to dealing with nontoxic nutrients, elaborate attempts are made to convert theoretical dangers into real ones. In sharp contrast, real therapeutic effectiveness is downgraded on theoretical reasons.

The fact that a single dose of 4 g of ascorbic acid increases excretion of uric acid and that 8 g per days does the same over a period of time ought to be a cause for rejoicing since it suggests that a new treatment for gout is possible. The modern treatment for gout calls for a reduction of serum uric acid levels. In fact these authors in a personal communication to AH had thought of this, but concluded that because of the large amount required it would be no cheaper than standard uricosuric drugs. But there is no reference whatever in this paper to the possible benefit and instead we are warned that "diminution in the serum uric acid may precipitate acute gouty arthritis in predisposed individuals."

One of us (AH) has used doses of ascorbic acid from 1½ to over 10 g per day on perhaps several thousand patients since 1952. Never has there been a single case of gout precipitated in any individual. Two were patients who now and then suffered gouty attacks before they started on ascorbic acid and after, but there was no increase in frequency. We would therefore conclude that the real probability of ascorbic acid inducing gouty attacks must be much less, if it occurs at all, than the natural incidence. When the first case appears where it is shown that the gout has been caused by ascorbic acid, then it will be time to look at it as a potential hazard.

In the biased nomenclature used in their "Discussion" on page 387, the authors speak of "chronic administration of 8 g of ascorbic acid per day." What they consider as "chronic" only happens to be a period of eight days, but even in this short time the serum uric acid levels were reduced about 30 percent from the starting values. What would have happened to the serum uric acid levels if the ascorbate administration was really "chronic" and continued throughout the subject's entire lifetime? Besides eliminating the chronic subclinical scurvy that afflicts all who are not taking many grams of ascorbate daily, its long-term uricosuric effect may have a very salutary action in preventing gout. The end product of purine metabolism in humans, uric acid, is different from most other mammals' because of the genetic lack of the enzyme uricase in Man. This is the enzyme that converts the rather insoluble uric acid into the more soluble allantoin. Research should be started to determine whether the chronic daily use of megadoses of ascorbate can catalyze the nonenzymatic transformation of uric acid to allantoin in Man. If it can, then the uric acid–stone formation problems would be solved.

In another ascorbic acid study, Norkus and Rosso (1975) examined the idea that high intake in pregnant guinea pigs would make the offspring more vulnerable to scurvy when placed upon a scorbutic diet.

Control group animals were given 25 mg of ascorbic acid daily (in human terms 3,500 mg per 70 kg human, assuming the experimental guinea pigs weighed about 500 g). They calculated that 300 mg per kg in the guinea pig is equivalent to 1,500 mg per human because there is a faster turnover in the guinea pig.

The ascorbic acid was added to the feed. They do not say how frequently the animals were fed, but it is logical to assume that they ate ad libitum, i.e., nibbled throughout the day as do rodents when food is freely available to them.

From Day 11 after birth the pups were caged individually and weaned onto the ascorbic acid-free diet. They were weighed and examined every third day for physical signs of scurvy. This was not done double blind. Once signs appeared they were examined every day.

As one would expect, the animals with higher ascorbic

acid levels metabolized more as measured by radioactive CO_2 release studies.

There was no difference between the groups in weight gain, but animals from high ascorbic acid mothers developed scurvy about four days earlier—in about 18 days compared to about 22 days for the other pups. The variation was four times as great for the first group, i.e., 0.96 compared to 0.21 S.E. for control group. Four of the nine high ascorbic acid group developed scurvy in about 22 days.

The high ascorbic acid group died in about 22 days compared to the control group which died in about 31 days.

On the basis of this work Norkus et al. concluded that "although one can not directly extrapolate these results to the human, because of different modes of ascorbic acid catabolism in guinea pig and Man, the results clearly support Cochrane's hypothesis that an ascorbic acid dependency in the young could be induced by exposure to high levels of this vitamin in utero." They then advise "massive doses of ascorbic acid during pregnancy should be discouraged."

The emphasis in their conclusion is wrong. In our view these experiments with guinea pigs suffer from the following methodological errors: the control group also received massive doses of ascorbic acid. It is amazing that modern diets for guinea pigs include daily doses of ascorbic acid in the range which we have been recommending. The usual megadoses for human adults are from 3 to 20 g per day, and only for severe stresses and deadly diseases such as viremias, cancer, and so on are doses larger than these used. The authors state that 300 mg per kg per guinea pig is equivalent to 1,500 mg per human adult, so why in designing their experimental protocol did they not use the guinea pig equivalent of the human RDA of 45 mg ascorbate per day for their control group, which calculates to 9 mg per kg? The weights of the guinea pigs were not given; if we assume they were closer to 500 g than a kilogram, then each control pig should be receiving 4.5 mg ascorbate per day instead of the 25 mg given. Did they use over 500 percent more than the RDA equivalent because they realized that the guinea pig mothers and pups may not have survived the stresses of pregnancy and birth on the bare subsistence levels recommended for humans?

Norkus et al. completely disregard the clinical work of Klenner (1971) in over 2,500 cases of human pregnancy and childbirth, in which the mothers were given throughout pregnancy, labor, and postpartum, 4 to 15 g ascorbate daily. Most also received a booster I.V. shot of 10 g of ascorbate on entering the hospital for labor. This resulted in great clinical benefits in avoiding the usual clinical problems of maternal health and labor and produced exceedingly robust healthy babies. . . .

In the discussion following the presentation of the Norkus et al. paper at the New York Academy of Sciences conference, Dr. C. W. M. Wilson of Dublin, Ireland, commented in part, "However, to draw such a conclusion for human beings seems completely wrong, because when a mother produces a child she does not deliberately expose him to scurvy by stopping ascorbic acid intake. . . ."

The authors of all these three highly critical reports still do not realize that in scurvy we are not dealing with a simple nutritional disturbance, but with a potentially fatal genetic liver-enzyme disease, Hypoascorbemia, whose terminal sequelae are what Medicine now regards as "scurvy." The terminal symptoms can be allayed by the RDA of 45 mg of ascorbate, but this is far too little to fully correct this human genetic defect. The RDA leaves victim suffering from chronic subclinical scurvy throughout life and is our most widespread disease (Stone, 1972b). To fully correct for this genetic defect requires amounts of ascorbate similar to that normally produced in the livers of other mammals each day. On a 70 kg body weight basis, this is in the range of 10 to 20 g per day (Chatterjee, 1973), so for humans this is not a "high" intake, but is the "normal" intake.

REFERENCES

Hoffer, A., "Ascorbic Acid and Toxicity," *New England Journal of Medicine,* vol. 285, p. 635, 1971.

Stich, H. F., Karim, J., Koropatnick, J., and Lo, L.,

"Mutagenic Action of Ascorbic Acid," *Nature,* vol. 260, pp. 722–724, 1976.

Stone, I., "The Natural History of Ascorbic Acid in the Evolution of the Mammals and Primates and its Significance for Present-Day Man," *Journal of Orthomolecular Psychiatry 1,* Nos. 2–3, pp. 82–89, 1972.

Subramanian, N., et al., "Detoxication of Histamines with Ascorbic Acid," *Biochemical Pharmacology,* vol. 22, pp. 1671–1673, 1973.

Nelson, M. M., and Forfar, J. O., "Association Between Drugs Administered During Pregnancy and Congenital Abnormalities of the Fetus," *British Medical Journal,* vol. 1, pp. 523–527, 1971.

Stone, I., *The Healing Factor* (New York: Grosset and Dunlap, 1972), pp. 87–88.

Stein, H. B., Hasan, A., and Fox, I. H., "Ascorbic Acid–Induced Uricosuira. A Consequence of Megavitamin Therapy," *Annals of Internal Medicine,* vol. 84, pp. 385–388, 1976.

Norkus, E. P., and Rosso, P., "Changes in Ascorbic Acid Metabolism of the Offspring Following High Maternal Intake of this Vitamin in the Pregnant Guinea Pig," *Annals of the New York Academy of Science,* vol. 258, pp. 401–409, 1975.

Klenner, F. R., "Observations on the Dose and Administration of Ascorbic Acid when Employed Beyond the Range of a Vitamin in Human Pathology," *Journal of Applied Nutrition,* vol. 23, pp. 61–87, 1971.

Stone, I., "Hypoascorbemia, our Most Widespread Disease," *National Health Federation Bulletin,* vol. 18, no. 10, pp. 6–7, 1972b.

Chatterjee, I. B., "Evolution and the Biosynthesis of Ascorbic Acid," *Science,* vol. 182, pp. 1271–1272, 1973.

25

You and Your Doctor

I know you will get flak when you ask most doctors to use massive amounts of vitamin C to treat cancer. I know because I once shared their views about new treatments and especially about nutritional treatments that were unfamiliar to me.

Let me help you understand doctors.

First, you must remember that doctors have been trained to be gods. They are supposed to know everything about the diagnosis and treatment of human illness. Most of them are well trained in everything except nutrition, in my present view the single most important aspect of prevention and treatment of illness.

Even if the doctor doesn't know everything, he has usually succumbed to the delusion that he knows everything. Sick people come to him and then get better. They might get better in *spite* of him instead of *because* of him; still, he takes the credit and stores it away in a little secret place in his heart, where the collection gradually grows larger and larger, totally convincing him that he is a great healer.

Your doctor needs the delusion that he is a Great Healer, otherwise he would worry himself sick dealing with matters of life and death day after day, making hundreds of decisions, any one of which could cost a human life if it is proved wrong.

Gods cannot stop every minute to wonder if they're doing the right thing.

Also, your doctor needs the delusion that he is a Great Healer to protect him when a patient dies. Every doctor loses patients. The doctor, to protect his sanity, must believe he is a Great Healer who did everything possible to save the patient. Otherwise he would be overcome with feelings of doubt and guilt.

So you are going to say to the Great Healer (who, chances are, knows very little about nutrition or vitamin C):

"I want vitamin C for my cancer."

What kind of reaction do you expect?

Right.

If he is the Great Healer and knows nothing about vitamin C for the treatment of cancer, he will be forced to damn it; otherwise his delusion will be shaken.

"If I don't know anything about the vitamin C treatment for cancer it must not be any good" is what he would like to say to you.

He would also like to remind you that he is the Great Healer and you shouldn't bother him about the nonsense you read in ladies' magazines and popular medical books.

But he won't be honest with you and tell you he doesn't know. He can't afford to be honest with you. It would crack his façade of omnipotence.

Instead, he'll say: "It hasn't been proven yet" or "There are reports of kidney stones from vitamin C."

The patient's dying of cancer and he's talking about kidney stones!

Or he might say: "In high doses I would be afraid the vitamin would clog your kidneys."

All these rebuttals, and any others that he might come up with, are nonsense.

Give him this book to read. If you get nowhere with your doctor, then you'll need to change doctors.

More on Understanding Doctors

Having read this far, you already understand a few things abut doctors. There are other things you need to know, however.

Medicine is one of the most conservative fields of learning. The old saying is that to introduce a new concept to the medical profession you simply have to wait for the old generation of doctors to die off.

When Harvey stated that blood circulated, his fellow doctors tried to kick him out of the medical society.

When Semmelweis told the medical profession they were infecting women by going straight from autopsies to the delivery room without changing their clothes or washing their hands, his colleagues ostracized him, and he spent the last years of his life wandering around the streets of Vienna telling people that doctors were killing their patients. A generation later, when bacteria were discovered, the medical profession nodded its collective head and said, yes, it looked as if Semmelweis had been right all along.

When the electroencephalogram came along, the profession called it a quack electrical device. Now almost every hospital has one.

That's about where the profession as a whole stands on new ideas.

Now as to the makeup of the individual doctor.

All of you have read how difficult it is to get into medical school. Believe me, it is one of the great contests of our society. You need to have a close to a straight A average to get in. Not only that, you've got to give evidence that you have more than academic ability. It helps to spend a summer working as an orderly in a mental hospital or shooting the rapids in a canoe in Colorado.

Those of us with psychiatric training know that medical students and doctors tend to have what we call obsessive-compulsive personalities. This is a scientific way of saying that many of them are quite rigid. It's quite difficult to get into med school if you aren't rigid. I know. I used to be that way myself, and recovered only with great difficulty.

For example, I went from a small, third-rate high school to Duke University, where I had to compete with boys from some of the best private schools in the world. I had to put my nose to the grindstone. During my first year in college I didn't even have a date. There wasn't time. My mornings were spent in classrooms. Laboratory work took up the afternoons, and my evenings were spent studying in the library. I would go to the library right after supper. (It was noisy in the dorms. The non-pre-med students were having fun bowling in the halls with empty beer cans.) In the library I would study fifty-five minutes straight, then walk out into the hall, stretch, get a drink of water and return for another fifty-five minutes, and on and on until the library closed—not now and then, but night after night, week after week, year after year.

Because of poor nutrition, I was sick half the time with colds and flu and depression. Looking back, I don't know how I did it.

But I'll tell you one thing, I paid my dues, and it doesn't make me feel guilty to be one of New York's highest-priced doctors.

Anyway, to leave my sad early life and get back to the point I was making . . . Doctors tend to be rigid people who practice medicine by the book while looking neither to the right nor to the left.

You know the doctors in your area. If you want one to treat you with a new method like vitamin C, go to one who has loosened up since medical school. Some of them are mellow. Some of them get secure enough to be able to admit that they don't know everything. Sometimes a younger doctor will be more open to a novel approach.

Don't bother trying to change the mind of a rigid doctor. No one ever has.

There's a third problem your doctor has with new ideas, especially those involving nutrition: fear of reprisal by his colleagues. It is a very real problem for doctors. If they don't stay in step, their narrow world might start closing in on them. Can you blame them? Who wants to lose his friends and his pocketbook?

So if your doctor won't help you, shop around.

The society listed below counts among its members doctors who are interested in and knowledgeable about the practical aspects of nutrition. I suspect many of them would be willing to give you vitamin C for cancer. You could write for a list of members.

International College of Applied Nutrition
P.O. Box 386
La Habra, California 90631

V

What I Believe

26

Conclusions

Today patients are better informed than ever about the workings of their bodies and the treatments they need when things don't go well. More and more patients are demanding that their doctors fully inform them about their condition and that they be given a voice in decisions made by physicians.

Some doctors find all this a nuisance. "Just do what I tell you and let me worry about things," many doctors want to tell their patients.

It's easier that way. Issuing commands saves time. It also saves wear and tear on the doctor. The more people he must relate to in depth during the course of a day, the tireder he's going to be at night.

Still, it's the patient's body and the patient's life that's at stake. Usually patients aren't stupid. They have a right to know.

DOCTORS ARE NOT ALWAYS HONEST

Doctors are not always honest with patients, especially about cancer.

"Don't tell Dad he has cancer," the family sometimes says to the doctor, conspiring in the veil of deception.

Personally, I don't want to be treated as an infant, and I don't think other people want that either. If I have pneumonia or tuberculosis or leprosy or cancer (or even an ingrown toenail, for that matter), I want to know all the facts so I can continue planning my life. Who can plan his life without knowing the facts?

I tell all patients the truth, the whole truth, and nothing but the truth. Partly I do it because that's the way I want to be treated. It's the only way of showing proper respect for a patient's adult intelligence. Besides, I'm too busy to remember lies. If I lied to every patient I would stumble sooner or later and the patient would learn that I had been lying. I won't see a patient that the family wants to "protect" from the facts.

Many doctors are not honest with patients suffering from cancer. They may tell the patient he has cancer, but then they twist the facts around.

Mrs. Nay, for example, told me that her doctors said she had about a 90 percent chance of living with chemotherapy. That simply isn't true. With very vigorous treatment for two years, she had at least a 30 percent chance of living a few years. How many, no one knows.

Later, when her cancer showed a progression, she was told that her chances were "very good" if she started chemotherapy again. When I talked with her doctor, he told me her chances were 5 percent, which I don't consider "very good."

I saw a patient the other day who had had breast surgery for cancer. Her doctor told her the chances were "98 percent that we have gotten out all the cancer" but they wanted to start her on chemotherapy "just to make sure." This was probably his way of telling her that the cancer had spread and she had better start chemotherapy. He was also not being honest when he said the chemotherapy would make sure.

YOU NEED THE FACTS

The best way to get the facts out of your doctor is to sit him down in private and level with him. Tell him you can't plan your life (or your death) unless you know all the raw facts. Tell him you are the type of person who needs to know and that he will be doing you no favor by withholding facts. Tell him you want a photocopy of your hospital records, including the pathology report. If necessary, take the records to a second doctor, tell him the same thing, and compare the conclusions given by the two doctors.

Oncologists, and doctors in general who deal with cancer, are incurably optimistic people. I suppose they must be, otherwise they would blow their brains out, surrounded as they are day after day with maimed and dying cancer patients. I suppose their optimism may sometimes reach unrealistic heights and what amounts to wishes is passed on to patients as facts.

At any rate, in this chapter I have tried to level with you as much as possible. Since you, as a patient suffering from cancer, are going to be called upon to participate in making decisions about the kind of treatment you receive, you need these facts.

Remember, however, that in the world of medicine there are few absolutes. For example, when I was a medical student at Duke I was taught that you should not transfuse a patient with a bleeding ulcer. When I went to the University of Chicago I was taught that you always transfused a patient with a bleeding ulcer.

Let me start on the firmest ground possible, however, and later move from there into the world opinion.

SURGERY

If a patient has cancer that can be surgically removed, then it usually should be taken out.

A couple of exceptions to this rule occur to me.

For example, early cancer of the prostate gland can usually be treated satisfactorily with irradiation. Surgical removal of the gland would probably leave the patient impotent.

Another possible exception is cancer of the skin, especially if the cancer is on the face, where surgery would be disfiguring. Usually skin cancers can be treated very satisfactorily with irradiation or chemotherapy. Several of us have had very good results by treating it with a combination of vitamin C by mouth and vitamin C ointment, together with vitamin A and other vitamins and minerals by mouth.

TERMINAL CANCER

If a patient has terminal cancer then surely he should be given vitamin C in massive amounts. There is not much to lose and a lot to gain. Diet and other vitamins and minerals should not be neglected.

CHEMOTHERAPY

These Are Best Bets for Chemotherapy (50 Percent or More Long-term Survival)

1. If the patient is suffering from acute childhood lymphocytic leukemia, then he should have chemotherapy.
2. If the patient has advanced Hodgkin's disease or one of the lymphomas, then he should have chemotherapy.
3. If the patient is a young man and has a testicular tumor, he should have chemotherapy and X-ray therapy, since the four- to 5-year survival in this disease has now gone up to about 90 percent.
4. Wilms' tumor, a relatively rare form of cancer that occurs in children, if treated vigorously with surgery, irradiation, and chemotherapy, has approximately an 80 percent long-term survival rate.
5. The chemotherapists speak of an 85 to 90 percent cure rate in a rare type of uterine cancer known as choriocarcinoma.
6. Burkitt's tumor, common in Africa, has a long-term survival rate of about 50 percent when treated with chemotherapy.
7. A muscular form of cancer called embryonal

rhabdomyosarcoma has a good long-term cure rate with chemotherapy.

8. Ewing's sarcoma, a form of bone cancer, is now above the 50 percent mark when surgery, X ray, and chemotherapy are all used.

9. With combined therapy, including chemotherapy, retinoblastomas (a form of eye cancer) are responding above the 50 percent mark.

10. Many skin cancers also respond well to chemotherapy.

When oncologists use the word *cure,* they may or may not mean what they say. Chemotherapeutic treatment of cancer is so new that oncologists are often not absolutely sure of their long-term survival rates. Often when they say cure they mean "five-year cure," which is to say that after a five-year interval the patient is apparently free of cancer. Some cancers (the breast cancers are notorious for this) may stay dormant for ten, fifteen, or even twenty years and then suddenly reappear.

But a 50 percent or better five-year cure rate is certainly a respectable figure. I think if I had one of the disorders listed above, I would opt for chemotherapy.

At the same time, I would follow a proper diet, take my vitamins and minerals, and down as much vitamin C as my system would tolerate. Generally speaking, the adverse symptoms from chemotherapy are lessened by the use of vitamin C in massive amounts, especially when used in conjunction with the other vitamins and minerals.

If chemotherapy makes one very sick for several years, it's probably worth putting up with it for 50–50 odds.

All my life I've tried to play the right odds. By that I mean I have treated patients by deciding what the odds were for harming the patient and what the odds were for helping the patient. Whether you are a doctor or a stockbroker, you've got to play the odds.

Once the odds for chemotherapy's producing a five-year cure rate go below 50–50, I quickly begin losing interest. The diseases discussed below fall into the long odds category.

Unfortunately, the forms of cancer with excellent chemotherapeutic results (50 percent cure rate or better) make up only about 15 percent of the total cancer seen. That is why the critics of chemotherapy point out that this new specialty has added very little to the over-all cure rate of cancer, and especially small amounts when one considers the great sums of money spent developing this branch of medicine.

Moderately Successful Cure Rates

Rosemary Nay, the patient discussed in the first and second chapters, was suffering from an oat cell carcinoma of the lung, one of the most deadly forms of cancer. The average patient is dead three or four months after the diagnosis is made. Surgery is of no help, and X-ray has little to offer.

Now, with very vigorous treatment, including the use of the highly toxic cis-platinum, about 30 percent of these patients are having long-term survival. In this case long-term survival is a somewhat ambiguous term. Generally it means a few years. The treatment hasn't been around long enough to speak clearly about five-year cures. At any rate, many patients with this diagnosis are definitely living longer than they did without the treatment.

But to achieve any significant increase in life span, chemotherapeutic treatment must be extremely vigorous and must go on for two years.

Most of the patients feel like walking dead while taking this 70–30 gamble.

We can never say absolutely what we would do in a given situation, but, knowing what I do now, I don't think I would take cis-platinum for any form of cancer with a less than 50–50 chance of cure. I might not take it even for those odds. The prospect of being deathly sick for two years even for 50–50 odds doesn't exactly turn me on.

Remember, however, that it is possible that patients taking even such a toxic drug as cis-platinum would tolerate it well enough to avoid two years of misery if they had had an adequate nutritional program *prior* to starting the chemotherapy.

Dr. Saccoman, who has probably had more experience than anyone else in treating patients with massive amounts of vitamin C while they are undergoing chemotherapy, told me he finds patients generally do better when vitamin C and chemotherapy are given at the same time. When chemotherapy is given first, he has the distinct impression patients do not do as well on vitamin C therapy.

There are complications, however.

Patients must go in the hospital from time to time for vigorous treatment of an oat cell carcinoma. Unfortunately, the doctors handling these cases will probably not know enough about vitamin C to carry it out properly while the patient is hospitalized. In fact because they will not be familiar with this treatment, they will probably condemn it. It's easier to say a form of therapy is no good than it is to take the trouble to learn about it.

Nausea is another difficulty. The vigorous chemotherapy given patients with oat cell carcinoma produces a great deal of trouble with nausea and vomiting. This means patients will have difficulty taking the ascorbic acid by mouth. Because their chemotherapy medication is given by vein, they sometimes reach the point where the veins are scarred and it is difficult to get any medication at all by that route, including ascorbic acid.

I think there is an ideal solution to this problem, hit upon by the three Japanese doctors who first give the chemotherapeutic medication by vein, then allow normal saline solution to run into the vein for twenty minutes (to keep the blood in the needle from clotting and to avoid having to traumatize the vein by puncturing it again), then give ascorbic acid intravenously using the same needle.

In this country oncologists are generally not going to

want to do this. Not only are they unfamiliar with the technique, not to say mistrustful of it, but often they will not want their "protocols smeared" with vitamin C. That is to say many of them are engaged in clinical research. They hope to come up with concrete figures about the usefulness of the drug or combination of drugs they are using, and thus are loath to add another factor (ascorbic acid and nutritional supplements) which would change the whole setup of the research project.

Premenopausal breast cancer, like oat cell carcinoma, is now enjoying a fair rate of cure. But here again, the treatment must be vigorous, and not everyone will want to go through it for the odds offered.

Chemotherapy for Other Forms of Cancer?

Do you want to feel desperately ill for two years trying for odds of 5 percent? If you do, go right ahead. I personally think that's about as sensible as making water into the wind. But there may be a few exceptions to consider.

The other day, for example, I saw a seventy-two-year-old man who had a cancer of the bowel removed. The oncologist wants to give him two chemotherapy treatments just in case there was some unrecognized spread. I think it's a waste of time (to date, bowel cancer has responded very poorly to chemotherapy) and might possibly be harmful, since it might lower the patient's natural resistance. However, I don't think two treatments is a very big deal one way or the other.

I have another patient who illustrates an interesting point. This man had an enlarged lymph node which was removed and examined. The pathologist reported that there was cancer in the node which had come from some other site. In other words, this was a metastatic lesion. Despite an extensive workup, his doctors were unable to find the primary site. Apparently his body had killed off the cancer where it had originally started.

This patient is given chemotherapy in a doctor's office every two weeks. He feels slightly tired and out of sorts for two or three days following the therapy, but otherwise gets along very well. He is able to take large amounts of vitamin C by mouth.

I suspect the chemotherapy is not doing anything to prolong this man's life. Since his doctors don't even know what kind of cancer they're dealing with, it is impossible to choose the drug most likely to help. But feeling a little off for two days every two weeks is not a very big imposition. The patient works full time and carries on a normal life.

No Chemotherapy Here

Some patients are absolutely unable to take chemotherapy. They may be allergic to the drug used. When a different drug is tried they may be allergic to that one also.

I had a patient consult me the other day who presented an interesting problem. This woman had been bothered on and off by colitis all her life. Last spring she had a breast amputated which showed cancer. The cancer had spread to two lymph nodes.

She was given two chemotherapy treatments at Memorial Sloan-Kettering, with the following results:

1. She developed diarrhea—up to forty liquid stools a day.
2. She began bleeding from her bowel.
3. She became suicidally depressed.
4. An all-engulfing fatigue descended upon her.
5. She developed severe pains in her bones.
6. Severe persistent headaches began.

At this point Memorial told her to leave off treatment and return in one month. She did not return. This patient has chosen to take the vitamin C treatment.

Who can blame her?

One other point I made with the patient, however. It is possible that after we get her in good nutritional shape and on large doses of vitamin C she might be able to handle the chemotherapy better. I told her she should seriously consider having one more try at chemotherapy after we've worked with her for about a month.

A trial at chemotherapy is often advisable. If you don't like it, you can always stop.

Also, a trial of a few weeks will often tell an oncologist whether a given chemical combination will be helpful in shrinking your tumor.

Please note well: I am not against chemotherapy. I am not competing with it for patients. I think there is a place for chemotherapy, a place for vitamin C therapy, and a place where they should be combined.

And there's always a place for a little common sense on everyone's part.

HORMONE THERAPY

As an intern at the University of Chicago in 1945, I spent a part of my year working with Dr. Charles Huggins, the urologist who discovered that removing the testicles and administering female sex hormones would prolong the lives of patients with cancer of the prostate. On his service we were busy cutting off testicles and administering diethylstilbestrol to men with prostatic cancer. (Huggins's work won him a Nobel prize for medicine in 1966.)

Time has proven Huggins's work to be valuable. If I had cancer of the prostate I would certainly consider having an orchidectomy and giving female sex hormones a try.

Sometimes the hormones cause men to have a change of personality. They may become more passive, and lose their sex drive. Sometimes the hormones make men depressed. If the depression cannot be handled satisfactorily with a proper diet and nutritional supplements (as outlined in this book in my chapters on diet and nutrition), then an alternate treatment should be considered. There is evidence that female sex hormones increase the incidence of coronary artery disease in men.

Most men can tolerate the hormones without any unreasonable change in their psychic life. Eighty percent of the patients have their lives prolonged two or three years. Any procedure which can accomplish that at a small price is certainly worth it.

Many non-urologists do not feel that removing the patient's testicles is helpful except the urologist.

Many surgeons think that it is worthwhile removing the ovaries of premenopausal women with breast cancer. Sometimes women with breast cancer are given testosterone, the male sex hormone, to slow the tumor growth. This hormone may have a masculinizing effect on women, giving them deep voices, causing excessive hair to grow on their faces and on other parts of their bodies, and making their muscles larger. Sometimes the greatest problem that comes from giving testosterone to women is sexual stimulation. When a sixty-year-old suddenly turns passionate and wants to make love twice a day, she may have trouble finding a partner to accommodate her needs.

Since testosterone may stimulate the appetite and act as a tonic in general, it is sometimes given to cancer patients in an attempt to get them to eat more.

Testosterone should never be given to men suffering from prostatic cancer.

X-RAY THERAPY

X-ray therapy comes in the form of what is traditionally called X-ray therapy (produced by an X-ray machine) or from radium or cobalt irradiation. These approaches are especially effective in treating several types of cancer. X-ray therapy does produce some unpleasant side effects, but they are usually mild compared to illness produced by chemotherapy.

Early Hodgkin's disease is very effectively treated with large doses of X ray.

Early prostatic cancer often responds quite well to

radiation. Because there is much less likelihood of the depression and impotence that go with hormone therapy, many patients choose this form of treatment.

In treating retinoblastoma (a type of eye cancer) in children the results are often highly satisfactory.

Early cancer of the larynx (the voice box) can usually be treated effectively with radiation. This method of therapy (unlike surgery) will leave the patient with the ability to speak.

Cancers in the nasopharynx (the upper part of the throat) are effectively treated with X ray.

Skin cancer often responds well to some form of irradiation.

The National Cancer Institute has reported that whole-body irradiation of patients with chronic lymphocytic leukemia has resulted in a doubling of their life expectancy. One in 3 patients has had long-term survival with this type of therapy.

After reading the successes listed above, the average reader might conclude that X-ray therapy just about has the cancer problem licked. Not so. The list does not include a high percentage of the total number of cancers. You don't see the big killers (percentage wise), such as cancer of the breast, lung cancers, and cancers of the gastrointestinal tract.

Most readers are aware that X-ray therapy in one form or another is used to treat almost every form of cancer. The treatment is usually palliative. That is to say, the therapy may make the tumors shrink temporarily or may reduce bone pain when the cancer has spread.

Proper nutritional therapy, especially when it includes large amounts of vitamin C, usually reduces the side effects of irradiation therapy.

VITAMIN C THERAPY FOR CANCER

Here are my conclusions about the use of Vitamin C to treat cancer:

1. There is something about vitamin C that is

deadly to cancer cells. This has been demonstrated in the test tube.

2. From three different sources we have clear-cut evidence that vitamin C ointment is very effective for curing skin cancer. At a medical meeting in the spring of 1978 in Palm Springs, one doctor reported that he routinely cured even advanced skin cancer with vitamin C ointment. Dr. Archie Kalokerinos of Mosman, New South Wales, Australia, told me he had excellent results with the use of vitamin C ointment in the treatment of skin cancers. I have had three patients with biopsy-proven early skin cancer who experienced rapid disappearance of their cancers after using vitamin C ointment.

There is no doubt in my mind that I would use vitamin C ointment if I developed skin cancer. In the unlikely event that it was not shrinking in a month's time, then I would turn to chemotherapy or irradiation treatment.

3. No matter what kind of treatment I chose for my cancer, I would want good nutritional therapy, including massive amounts of vitamin C. Cameron and Pauling have demonstrated that it helps in a large variety of cancers. Their findings have been confirmed by Dr. Saccoman, in San Diego, by Drs. Kalokerinos and Lent, in Australia, and by me.

4. Massive amounts of vitamin C reduce the unpleasant side effects from X-ray therapy and chemotherapy. It may well make them work more effectively.

5. Vitamin C in large amounts generally increases the patients' feeling of well-being a great deal. They get out of bed. They take an interest in life again. They move back into the land of the living.

6. Everyone using vitamin C in the treatment of cancer reports that tumors are shrunk by the use of this vitamin. This represents a palliative effect from the vitamin. Although this effect may not be all we want, it is much the same effect that is obtained in the treatment of the vast majority of patients with the use of X-ray and chemotherapy. Vitamin C might well

replace these two therapies when they are used for palliative effects.

7. I know of only one doctor (who wishes to remain anonymous) who flatly states that he cures generalized cancer with vitamin C. It is true that he uses far more of the vitamin than anyone else. He recommends that the patient take as much as possible by mouth. In addition, he recommends 60 grams to be given intravenously eighty times within one hundred days.

Will this cure cancer? I don't know, but I plan to find out. I am now using such a treatment on a patient with disseminated cancer. This patient is also taking 48 grams a day by mouth. This means she will have 9,600 grams (almost 10,000,000 milligrams) during this hundred-day period.

Cameron and Pauling report that one patient with advanced lymphoma responded with a clearing of the tumors within two weeks when given only 10 grams of vitamin C daily. He relapsed when he later left off the vitamin. When he started it again, the cancer cleared up once more, though more slowly. The patient now continues his vitamin C and continues his complete remission. Is the patient cured? No one knows for sure, but his cancer is certainly totally controlled by the vitamin C.

8. Here are the success rates as reported by Cameron and Pauling:

Terminally ill patients with these forms of cancer when given 10 grams of vitamin C daily lived five to ten times as long as untreated controls:

> Colon (13 cases)
> Leukemia (1 case)
> Lymphoma (2 cases)
> Leiomyosarcoma (1 case)
> Carcinoid (1 case)
> Bronchus (15 cases)

It is especially interesting that the above list includes carcinoma of the colon and lung cancer, since from a statistical standpoint these are two of the biggest killers and two types of cancer that respond rather poorly to X-ray therapy and to chemotherapy.

The following types of cancer lived four to five times as long as the untreated controls:

> Breast (11 cases)
> Kidney (9 cases)
> Bladder (7 cases)
> Rectum (7 cases)

Patients with these types of cancer lived three times as long as the untreated controls:

> Pseudomyxoma (1 case)
> Stomach (12 cases)

These patients lived approximately two times as long:

> Ovary (6 cases)
> Pancreas (3 cases)
> Prostate (1 case)
> Gallbladder (2 cases)

Patients with this type of cancer lived no longer than the controls:

> Uterus (1 case)

Terminally ill patients with these forms of cancer did not live as long as the controls when given vitamin C at the 10 gram per day level:

> Fibrosarcoma (1 case)
> Testicle (1 case)
> Chondrosarcoma (1 case)
> Brain (1 case)

Where there are only a few cases involved the conclusions may or may not be valid.

My Final Conclusions

It's always risky saying in advance what you would do in a given situation. I have had to make life-or-death choices about my own health on two separate occasions, however, so the act of choosing is not unknown to me.

Ten years ago I had a coronary followed by anginal heart pain. I chose not to go with conventional medical treatments, which offered me a 50–50 chance for five-year survival. My choice turned out to be correct. To-day I am in excellent health, without any signs or symptoms of heart disease. I can run, walk fast against the wind on cold days, and otherwise carry on with my daily life without any chest pain.

Four years ago I developed a severe case of hepati-tis. I was told by a professor of medicine at Mount Sinai that the chances were 80–20 that I would live if I took cortisone. If I didn't take it, he said, the chances were 80–20 that I would die.

After giving it a try, I found that the cortisone inter-fered with my ability to write. I didn't care for this side effect. Also, I had the feeling that this steroid would adversely affect my cardiovascular system. I opted against steroid therapy and for nutritional ther-apy.

About two years ago I had a checkup by the same professor, who pronounced me free of all signs of liver damage.

I have done my best to impartially give you all the facts in order to help you reach your own conclusions. Now it's up to you to pick your horse and place your bets.

Don't forget, however, that it's possible to hedge your bet. You can often bet on nutritional therapy combined with surgery or with X ray or with chemo-therapy, or perhaps with all three.

ONE LAST WORD

We have long accepted the fact that the treatment of cancer is a team approach consisting of a surgeon and a therapeutic radiologist. During the past twenty-five years the oncologist has been added to the team.

Now it's time for another specialist to join these three: the medical nutritionist. A medical nutritionist has much to offer the cancer patient. Without his help, the patient with cancer will be getting second-class medical care.

If you would like another opinion about your condition, about acceptable forms of treatment and your prognosis, I would suggest you consult *The Merck Manual*, published by Merck Sharp & Dohme Research Laboratories in Rahway, New Jersey. In case you run across terms you don't understand, you might like to also have *Dorland's Pocket Medical Dictionary*, published by W. B. Saunders Company in Philadelphia.

Epilogue

It was early December, 1977, when Mrs. Nay sparked my interest in the vitamin C treatment of cancer. As I write this now, it's early August, 1978. Eight months have passed. Let me bring you up to date.

First, you remember that Mrs. Nay felt so bad on chemotherapy that she was unable to continue it. When she came to see me she said that her doctors at Memorial had told her she would be back begging for more chemotherapy by the end of the month. They were wrong. By the end of December, Mrs. Nay was feeling great.

In order to keep what follows in proper perspective, remember that Mrs. Nay is suffering from a form of lung cancer known as oat cell, a very deadly type. As a rule patients are dead three or four months after the diagnosis is established.

Mrs. Nay had a very good period from Christmas to the fourth of July. She worked regularly, bought a new house, went to parties, and led a normal life. She was happy and free of pain, and her strength was good.

A chest X ray in April showed she had some return of the cancer that had disappeared with chemotherapy.

Around the fourth of July the patient developed a sharp pain in her right chest. She thought she might have pulled a muscle while exercising. The pain soon disappeared, but we had her get another X ray, which showed some increase in the cancer, as well as a small amount of fluid in her right chest.

This was a crisis point for the patient and her husband. They had another conference with her oncologist, who advised that she be hospitalized for X-ray therapy and chemotherapy.

I encouraged the meeting and told Mrs. Nay that she might be able to tolerate the chemotherapy better now that she was on the vitamin C and other nutritional supplements. Once more she decided against X-ray treatment or chemotherapy.

Based on the reports of the doctor mentioned earlier (who wishes to remain anonymous) that he was curing cancer by giving as much vitamin C by mouth as patients could tolerate plus 60 grams of vitamin C intravenously eighty times within a hundred-day period, I decided to start Mrs. Nay on this program. The treatment began July 19, 1978.

Mrs Nay continues to do well. She has a slight cough but no pain. She continues working. The other day when she was walking up hill she found herself a bit tired, but by and large everything still goes well.

What will happen? Will she be like some of Cameron's patients, who have a good life until near the end and then suddenly go into a tailspin and die? Or will the massive amount of vitamin C cure her cancer?

I don't know. We can only continue the fight and hope for the best.

Whatever happens, I feel very strongly that Mrs. Nay's life has been greatly prolonged by the use of massive amounts of vitamin C (along with other nutrients), and certainly she has felt vastly better than before.

Appendices

Appendix A
Supplemental Ascorbate in the Supportive Treatment of Cancer: Prolongation of Survival Times in Terminal Human Cancer *

By Ewan Cameron and Linus Pauling

Abstract

Ascorbic acid metabolism is associated with a number of mechanisms known to be involved in host resistance to malignant disease. Cancer patients are significantly depleted of ascorbic acid, and in our opinion this demonstrable biochemical characteristic indicates a substantially increased requirement and utilization of this substance to potentiate these various host resistance factors.

The results of a clinical trial are presented in which 100 terminal cancer patients were given supplemental ascorbate as part of their routine management. Their progress is compared to that of 1000 similar patients treated identically, but who received no supplemental ascorbate. The mean survival time is more than 4.2 times as great for the ascorbate subjects (more than 210 days) as for the controls (50 days). Analysis of the survival-time curves indicate that deaths occur for about 90% of the ascorbate-treated patients at one-third the rate for the controls and that the other 10% have a much greater survival time, averaging more than 20 times that for the controls.

The results clearly indicate that this simple and safe form of medication is of definite value in the treatment of patients with advanced cancer.

There is increasing awareness that the progress of human cancer is determined to some extent by the natural

---

* Publication no. 63 from the Linus Pauling Institute of Science and Medicine. This is part I of a series.

Appeared in *Proceedings of the National Academy of Science U.S.A.*, vol. 73, pp. 3685–3689, October 1976, Medical Sciences.

resistance of the patient to his disease. Consequently there is growing recognition that improvement in the management of these patients could come from the development of practical supportive measures specifically designed to enhance host resistance to malignant invasive growth.

We have advanced arguments elsewhere indicating that one important factor in host resistance is the free availability of ascorbic acid.[1-3] These arguments as based upon the demonstration that cancer patients have a much greater requirement for this substance than normal healthy individuals, on the realization that ascorbic acid metabolism can be implicated in a number of mechanisms known to be involved in host resistance, and finally, and most convincingly, on the published evidence that ascorbic acid can sometimes produce quite dramatic remissions in advanced human cancer.[4, 5]

In this communication we present the results of a clinical trial in which 100 terminal cancer patients received supplemental ascorbate as their only definitive form of treatment and compare their progress with that of 1000 matched patients managed by the same clinicians in the same hospital who did not receive any ascorbate supplementation or any other definitive form of specific anticancer treatment.

Protocol

The study involved a treated group of 100 patients with terminal cancer of various kinds and a control group of 1000 untreated and matched patients. The treated group consists of 100 patients who began ascorbate treatment, as described by Cameron and Campbell [4] (usually 10 g/day, by intravenous infusion for about 10 days and orally thereafter), at the time in the progress of their disease when in the considered opinion of at least two independent clinicians the continuance of any conventional form of treatment would offer no further benefit. Fifty of the treated subjects are those described in ref. 4 and the other 50 were obtained by random selection from the alphabetical index of ascorbate-treated patients in Vale of Leven District General Hospital, where treatment of some terminal cancer patients with ascorbate has been under clinical trial since November 1971. We believe that the ascorbate-treated patients represent a random selection of all of the terminal patients in this hospital, even though no formal randomization process was used. In the random selection three patients were excluded because supplemental ascorbate had been deliberately discontinued by order of another physician, and five were excluded because matching controls could not be found for them. Patients suspected or known to have voluntarily discontinued ascorbate treatment have been retained in the group, as have those who died from some cause other than their cancer. No patient was excluded because of short survival time. Eighteen patients, marked with a plus sign in Table 1, were still alive on 10 August 1976, 16 of them clinically "well." These 100 cancer patients, given ascorbate from the presentation date in their illness when their disease process was recognized to be "untreatable" by any conventional method, comprise the treated group.

The control group was obtained by a random search of the case record index of similar patients treated by the same clinicians in Vale of Leven Hospital over the last 10 years. For each treated patient, 10 controls were found of the same sex, within 5 years of the same age, and who had suffered from cancer of the same primary organ and histological tumor type. These 1000 cancer patients comprise the control group.

The detailed case records of these 1000 were then analyzed quite independently by Dr. Frances Meuli, M.B., Ch.B. (Otago, New Zealand), whose established their presentation date of "untreatability" by such conventional standards as the establishment of inoperability at laparotomy, the abandonment of any definitive form of anticancer treatment, or the final date of admission for "terminal care." This presentation date of untreatability corresponds to the date when ascorbate supplementation was initiated in the treated group. Comparable survival times of the 10 matched controls could then be calculated. We accept that "the presentation date of untreatability" can be influenced by many factors in individual patients, but we contend that the use of 1000 controls managed by the same clinicians in the same hospital over the last 10 years provides a sound basis for this comparative study.

We record our thanks to Dr. Meuli for her unbiased and valuable contribution to this investigation.

Even though no formal process of randomization was carried out in the selection of our two groups, we believe that they come close to representing random subpopulations of the population of terminal cancer patients in Vale of Leven Hospital. There is some internal evidence in the data in Table 1 to support this conclusion.

A somewhat detailed description of the circumstances under which the study was made may be called for. Of the 375 beds in Vale of Leven Hospital, 100 are in the surgical unit, 50 in the medical unit, and 25 in the gynecological unit. The 100 beds in the surgical unit are in the administrative charge of Ewan Cameron, and 50 of them are in his complete clinical charge, the other 50 being in the charge of the second Consultant Surgeon of the Hospital. The two Consultant Surgeons are assisted by a changing group of four Surgical Registrars, who are qualified surgeons on assignment for terms of 6 or 12 months from one or another of the Glasgow teaching hospitals. They are assisted by residents and interns. Although some cancer patients are initially treated in the medical or gynecological unit, there is a tendency for cases of advanced cancer of all kinds except leukemia and some rare childhood cancers, which are dealt with in a pediatric hospital in Glasgow, to gravitate into the surgical unit, in total probably 90% of all cases of cancer in the Loch Lomondside area.

All of the patients are treated initially in a perfectly conventional way, by operation, use of radiotherapy, and administration of hormones and cytotoxic substances. For example all of the 11 breast-cancer patients in the ascorbate-treated group, with the exception of one who first presented in a grossly advanced state, had already had mastectomy and radiotherapy and all, including the exception, had been given hormones, sometimes with considerable benefit; but all had relapsed by the time ascorbate supplementation was commenced, and it seemed clear that their tumors were escaping from hormonal control. Similarly, all of the seven bladder-cancer patients in the ascorbate-treated group, with one exception because of her frailty, had received megavoltage irradiation and several had had a partial cystectomy (one total) before ascorbate treatment was commenced when it seemed that these standard procedures had failed.

Treatment of terminal cancer patients with ascorbate was cautiously begun in November 1971, for reasons discussed in our earlier papers,[1, 2] and has been continued because it seemed to have some value.[4, 5] Once the practice had become locally established, the selection of a patient for treatment with ascorbate was often initiated by one of the younger surgeons (the Registrars), as they became familiar with the idea and convinced of its worth. The suggestion that ascorbate treatment be tried was made by Registrars less often during the first part of their 6 to 12 months' service than during the second part. For strong ethical reasons every patient in the ascorbate-treated group was examined and assessed independently by at least two physicians or surgeons (often more than two) who all agreed that the situation was "totally hopeless" and "quite untreatable" before ascorbate was commenced. More than 20 different Registrars were involved in this way in allocating patients to the ascorbate-treated group. No criterion was used, except agreed "untreatability."

As described above, selection of 10 matched patients for the control group for each patient of the ascorbate-treated group was made independently by Dr. Frances Meuli. For each ascorbate-treated patient she was given a sheet listing age, sex, primary tumor type, and a brief synopsis of the clinical state and extent of dissemination at the time ascorbate was commenced, but not the survival time. She searched for cases matching these cases as closely as possible, and assigned to each, from the case history, the time when the patient was classified as "untreatable." We believe that the procedure that was followed has not introduced any serious error, and that the ascorbate-treated group and the control group are in fact subpopulations of the population of "untreatable" patients selected in an essentially random manner.

Two hundred of the 1000 patients in the control group were completely contemporaneous with the ascorbate-treated patients. The mean survival time for these contemporaneous controls is 43.9 days, as compared with 52.4 days for the others (overlapping and historical). There

Table 1

Comparison of time of survival of 100 cancer patients who received ascorbic acid and 1000 matched patients with no treatment[a]

Case no.	Primary tumor type	Sex	Age	Survival time (days) — Ten matched controls: Individuals										Mean	Test case	Test case/ mean control (%)
1.	Stomach	F	61	12	41	5	29	85	124	8	54	21	36	38.5	121	314
2.	Stomach	M	69	8	6	3	9	4	26	8	114	15	14	20.7	12	58
3.	Stomach	F	62	15	1	72	19	19	27	35	99	76	111	47.4	9	19
4.	Stomach	F	66	4	87	7	11	3	13	12	6	34	35	21.2	18	85
5.	Stomach	M	42	8	1	74	358	9	84	14	16	16	128	70.8	258	368
6.	Stomach	M	79	45	4	12	1	9	6	12	130	4	11	23.4	43	184
7.	Stomach	M	76	22	19	12	9	14	7	15	3	5	14	12.0	142	1183
8.	Stomach	M	54	24	26	21	61	27	48	7	26	2	221	46.3	36	78
9.	Stomach	M	62	14	23	13	89	4	11	4	4	36	27	22.5	149+	622
10.	Stomach	F	69	6	19	55	2	21	8	53	11	103	17	29.5	182+	617
11.	Stomach	M	45	17	24	7	57	128	16	44	64	110	78	54.5	82	150
12.	Stomach	M	57	19	13	8	11	39	29	41	17	170	5	36.9	64	173
13.	Bronchus	M	74	16	56	29	27	67	41	25	26	6	40	33.3	39	117
14.	Bronchus	M	74	21	2	27	30	18	1	31	1	21	16	16.8	427	2542
15.	Bronchus	M	66	47	94	7	39	3	53	5	4	82	9	34.3	17	50
16.	Bronchus	M	52	35	4	70	21	126	8	46	272	39	75	69.6	460	661

No.	Tissue	Sex	Age													
17.	Bronchus	F	48	11	33	30	5	6	1	45	24	81	57	29.3	90	307
18.	Bronchus	F	64	7	1	26	13	71	14	4	30	103	2	27.1	187	690
19.	Bronchus	M	70	24	8	20	7	62	20	5	41	19	49	25.5	58	227
20.	Bronchus	M	78	32	19	39	40	24	21	43	103	2	21	34.4	52	151
21.	Bronchus	M	71	5	53	7	30	2	5	20	39	31	16	20.8	100	481
22.	Bronchus	M	70	3	2	33	24	25	35	25	62	2	63	27.4	200+	730
23.	Bronchus	M	39	42	31	74	5	88	45	28	3	15	70	40.1	42	105
24.	Bronchus	M	70	24	1	30	2	5	42	46	41	7	57	25.5	167	655
25.	Bronchus	M	70	8	34	29	24	5	4	32	129	20	51	40.7	33	81
26.	Esophagus	M	72	12	21	19	14	81	26	59	21	28	33	57.4	50	87
27.	Esophagus	F	80	2	29	6	45	48	24	13	238	56	2	46.3	43	93
28.	Colon	F	76	2	2	18	5	20	22	1	1	4	1	7.6	57	750
29.	Colon	F	58	56	39	31	15	9	11	8	10	6	62	24.7	32	130
30.	Colon	M	49	35	122	107	28	30	13	78	65	46	56	58.0	201	347
31.	Colon	M	69	48	9	7	15	30	90	26	94	38	15	37.3	1267	4343
32.	Colon	F	70	64	102	13	82	8	51	33	144	17	11	52.5	144	274
33.	Colon	F	68	9	15	40	11	17	217	163	59	18	38	38.5	170	442
34.	Colon	M	50	7	108	7	18	17	14	51	69	16	(32)	33.8	428	1266
35.	Colon	F	74	11	45	50	6	18	26	40	11	88	23	31.8	157+	494
36.	Colon	M	66	13	7	224	31	72	11	1	4	11	14	38.8	58	149
37.	Colon	F	76	23	129	8	63	60	21	28	3	15	70	43.8	123+	281
38.	Colon	F	56	24	1	30	2	5	42	46	41	7	57	25.5	861	3376
39.	Rectum	F	56	51	406	74	36	41	106	30	82	82	98	100.6	62	62
40.	Rectum	F	75	3	40	46	58	7	9	19	68	16	178	44.4	223	502
41.	Rectum	M	56	3	18	52	36	34	7	49	3	6	(13)	22.2	18	81
42.	Rectum	F	57	9	73	11	19	98	82	(184)	(97)	(89)	(47)	70.9	223	314

Case no.	Primary tumor type	Sex	Age	Individuals										Mean	Test case	Test case/ mean control (%)
43.	Rectum	M	68	11	11	91	47	18	23	4	13	79	84	38.1	140+	367
44.	Rectum	M	54	52	36	10	127	18	98	6	73	11	19	45.0	198	440
45.	Rectum	M	59	15	2	78	8	98	30	140	54	233	(14)	67.2	759	1129
46.	Ovary	F	49	36	5	117	29	31	22	101	140	94	73	64.8	226	349
47.	Ovary	F	68	41	39	18	37	67	3	91	40	6	13	35.5	33	93
48.	Ovary	F	49	53	15	38	122	68	33	841	18	21	40	124.9	183	146
49.	Ovary	F	67	19	36	22	2	10	32	48	132	21	97	41.9	240+	573
50.	Ovary	F	56	49	39	22	85	160	1	86	106	99	107	75.4	123+	163
51.	Breast	F	56	1	65	26	6	2	15	19	102	71	131	43.8	4	9
52.	Breast	F	57	3	28	15	4	14	16	14	48	61	15	21.8	22	101
53.	Breast	F	53	33	183	6	190	45	29	16	45	109	34	69.0	576	835
54.	Breast	F	66	22	12	94	55	7	38	2	10	76	12	102.8	342	333
55.	Breast	F	68	107	41	69	19	17	251	101	81	50	52	78.8	567	720
56.	Breast	F	53	8	2	2	42	31	17	96	231	42	20	49.1	86	175
57.	Breast	F	75	45	175	12	91	27	5	20	11	63	73	74.2	590	795
58.	Breast	F	74	12	2	35	6	18	33	30	107	85	47	37.5	8	21
59.	Breast	F	49	3	16	62	44	1	17	93	73	5	57	37.1	35	94
60.	Breast	F	50	31	29	28	40	265	14	31	24	104	229	82.6	1644+	1990
61.	Breast	F	53	105	73	193	159	8	127	126	167	71	42	107.1	173+	162
62.	Bladder	M	93	17	47	21	12	2	18	21	46	133	48	36.5	241	660
63.	Bladder	F	70	39	9	126	52	26	97	10	8	7	79	45.3	253	556
64.	Bladder	F	73	1	23	52	30	38	38	25	13	45	24	28.9	110	381

#	Site	Sex														
65.	Bladder	F	77	3	52	48	142	118	34	33	10	38	26	50.4	34	67
66.	Bladder	M	44	6	9	36	48	10	21	8	52	42	16	24.8	34	137
67.	Bladder	M	62	47	118	85	76	19	58	127	72	10	15	62.7	669+	1067
68.	Bladder	M	69	39	5	66	26	25	267	85	12	13	27	56.5	30	53
69.	Gallbladder	F	71	7	8	56	22	91	44	30	22	47	14	34.1	22	64
70.	Gallbladder	M	67	20	159	4	212	73	60	94	31	16	91	76.0	209	275
71.	Kidney (Ca)	F	71	6	2	17	83	81	55	14	114	60	106	53.8	176	327
72.	Kidney (Ca)	F	63	68	76	8	31	26	5	8	69	29	49	36.9	89	241
73.	Kidney (Ca)	F	51	16	82	27	41	65	29	8	125	(95)	(117)	60.6	147	243
74.	Kidney (Ca)	M	53	7	15	7	49	95	21	91	35	19	76	41.5	58	140
75.	Kidney (Ca)	M	55	15	13	12	16	45	48	89	95	6	83	42.2	659	1562
76.	Kidney (Ca)	M	73	25	11	209	19	30	198	31	7	30	50	61.0	293	480
77.	Kidney (Ca)	M	45	91	35	19	77	64	12	127	74	34	82	61.5	3	5
78.	Kidney (Pap)	M	69	67	74	(24)	(37)	87[b]	43[b]	21[b]	82[b]	14[b]	41[b]	49.0	24	49
79.	Kidney (Pap)	M	74	57	67	51	(491)	(127)	324	174	126[b]	179[b]	97[b]	169.3	1554+	918
80.	Lymphoma	M	40	144	41	53	29	16	20	41	279	302	103	102.8	1016+	988
81.	Lymphoma	M	65	28	68	51	56	117	138	10	36	51	142	69.7	82	118
82.	Prostate	M	47	24	14	22	23	101	53	157	123	16	80	82.3	166+	202
83.	Uterus	F	56	25	11	7	67	130	126	30	18	185	61	66.0	68	103
84.	Chondrosarcoma	M	63	20	25	3	17	136	17	31	23	19	157	44.8	9	20
85.	"Brain"	M	49	1	85	56	(187)	57	24	13	29	1	95	54.8	37	67
86.	Pancreas	M	77	11	25	19	38	91	78	13	41	40	94	45.0	317	704
87.	Pancreas	M	67	112	6	55	36	256	25	13	76	67	52	77.6	21	27
88.	Pancreas	F	60	11	42	23	49	57	69	91	253	89	59	77.4	16	21
89.	Fibrosarcoma	F	54	13	1	171	10	30	64	122	(9)	(25)	(17)	44.1	22	50
90.	Testicle	M	42	11	10	56	46	39	102	(101)	(19)	(29)	(87)	41.6	15	36

Case no.	Primary tumor type	Sex	Age	Individuals										Mean	Test case	Test case/ mean control (%)
91.	Pseudomyxoma	M	47	35	16	1	19	(37)	(27)	(12)	(15)	(87)	(162)	41.1	132	321
92.	Carcinoid	F	68	19	12	45	8	31	12	18	15	82	(38)	28.0	162+	579
93.	Leiomyosarcoma	F	32	31	74	66	(28)	(87)	(121)	[21]	[44]	[27]	[242]	74.1	453+	611
94.	Leukemia	F	59	6	36	183	6	36	32	44	36	112	63	55.4	430+	776
95.	Stomach	M	55	34	34	12	78	5	253	77	79	72	49	69.3	27	39
96.	Ovary	F	51	128	13	76	31	65	216	62	140	62	40	83.3	82	98
97.	Bronchus	M	69	92	30	90	160	43	147	32	20	135	125	87.4	31	35
98.	Bronchus	F	67	93	20	29	90	97	68	185	8	37	26	65.3	138	211
99.	Colon	M	77	8	69	80	14	30	9	57	68	14	21	37.0	15	40
100.	Colon	M	38	3	41	78	17	58	40	66	98	42	(80)	52.3	152+	291

^a The sign + following the survival time of the patients treated with ascorbic acid means that the patient was alive on August 10, 1976. Parentheses () indicate that the matched patient had the same sex, same kind of tumor, and same dissemination, but had an age difference greater than 5 years. Brackets [] indicate opposite sex, same tumor, same dissemination, age difference greater than 5 years. For kidney, Ca indicates carcinoma, Pap, papilloma.

^b Diffuse urinary tract papillomatosis. The test cases (78 and 79) had lesions in both kidney and bladder. The nine control cases indicated had tumors of identical histology, but their disease was confined to bladder mucosa.

has been no significant change in the treatment of patients with advanced cancer in Vale of Leven Hospital during the last 10 years, and the approximate equality of these values is not surprising.

The Results of the Study

The results of the study are given in Table 1 and summarized in Table 2, in which values for different kinds of cancer represented by six or more patients treated with ascorbate (60 or more controls) are shown. For each of the nine categories the ratio of average days of survival (ascorbate/controls) is greater than unity, the range being from 2.1 to 7.6, with ratio 4.16 for all 100 patients. The ratios are somewhat uncertain; for example, omitting the patient with longest survival in the colon group would decrease the ratio from 7.6 to 5.2. At the present time we cannot conclude that ascorbate has less value for one kind of cancer than for others. Our conclusion is that the administration of ascorbic acid in amounts of about 10 g/day to patients with advanced cancer leads to about a 4-fold increase in their life expectancy, in addition to an apparent improvement in the quality of life. This great increase in survival time results in part from the much larger numbers of the ascorbate patients than of the controls who live for long times, as is shown in Fig. 1. Sixteen percent of the patients treated with ascorbate acid survived for more than a year, 50 times the value for the controls (0.3%).

Statistical analysis shows that the null hypothesis that treatment with ascorbate has no benefit is to be rejected for each of the categories in Table 2. The results of a simple statistical test are given in the table. A reasonable dividing line, the average survival time for all the subjects, is given in column E, and the percentages exceeding this value are given in columns F and G. Column H contains the values of χ^2 obtained by a two-by-two calculation, and I gives the corresponding values of P (one-tailed). Similar values are obtained by nonparametric methods.

The fraction of survivors of the control group at time t is given to within about 2% by the exponential expression $\exp(-t/\tau)$. About 1.5% of the patients in this group live

349

Table 2

Ratios of average survival times for ascorbate patients and matched controls, with statistical significance

A	B (Days)	C (Days)	D	E (Days)	F (%)	G (%)	H	I
Bronchus (15)	136	38.5	3.53	47	47	8.7	24.5	$\ll 0.0001$
Colon (13)	282	37.0	7.61	59	54	20	7.63	< 0.003
Stomach (13)	98.9	37.9	2.61	43	46	17	6.41	< 0.006
Breast (11)	367	64.0	5.75	91	55	22	5.74	< 0.026
Kidney (9)	333	64.0	5.21	88	67	22	8.35	< 0.002
Bladder (7)	196	43.6	4.49	57	57	20	4.90	< 0.028
Rectum (7)	226	55.5	4.10	71	86	33	7.57	< 0.003
Ovary (6)	148	71.0	2.08	78	83	30	6.83	< 0.005
Others (19)	172	56.8	3.03	67	53	27	5.28	< 0.027
All (100)	209.6	50.4	4.16	65	60	25.7	55.02	$\ll 0.0001$

A, Type of cancer and, in parentheses, number of ascorbate patients. There are 10 matched controls for each ascorbic acid patient. B, Average days of survival for ascorbate patients. C, Average days of survival for controls. D, The ratio B/C. E, Average days of survival for all subjects in group. F, Percentage of ascorbate patients surviving longer than E. G, Percentage of controls surviving longer than E. H, Value of x^2 for F and G (two-by-two calculation). I, Corresponding value of P (one-tailed).

350

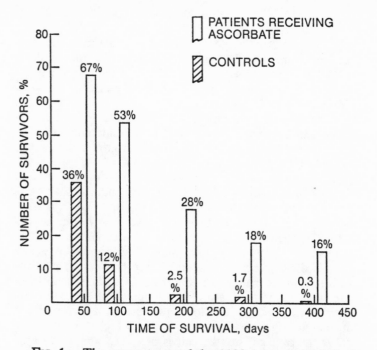

FIG. 1. The percentages of the 1000 controls (matched cancer patients) and the 100 patients treated with ascorbic acid (other treatment identical) who survived by the indicated number of days after being deemed "untreatable." The values at 200, 300, and 400 days for the patients receiving ascorbate are minimum values, corresponding to the date August 10, 1976, when 18% of these patients were still alive (none of the controls).

much longer than would be indicated by this expression. A very close approximation to the observed survival curve is given by the assumption that the control group consists of two populations. One consists of 985 patients with number of survivors at time t given by the expression $985 \exp(-t/\tau)$, in which τ has the value of 45.5 days. This expression corresponds to a constant mortality rate for this subgroup, and its validity suggests that for them a single random process, occurring with a probability independent of time, leads to death. This probability is 2.2% per day. For 14 of the 1000 control patients the survival time is indicated to lie between 200 and 500 days. The distribution suggests that for this subgroup two random events lead to death, but the number of subjects is too small to permit this possibility to be tested thoroughly. One other patient, who survived 841 days, may constitute a third subgroup.

A similar analysis of the survival curve for the ascorbate-treated group shows that a considerably smaller fraction, 90%, constitutes the principal group, with number of survivors at time t equal to $90 \exp(-t/\tau)$, τ equal to 125 days. For the remaining 10% the average survival time is greater than 970 days. (These numbers are uncertain because the number of ascorbate-treated patients is small, only 100, and 18 of them were alive on August 10, 1976, their survival times being greater than the values used in the calculation.) A simple interpretation of these facts is that the administration of ascorbate to the patients with terminal cancer has two effects. First, it increases the effectiveness of the natural mechanisms of resistance to such an extent as to lead to an increase by a factor of 2.7 in the average survival time for most of the patients; 2.7 is the ratio of the two values of τ, 125 and 45.5 days. Second, it has another effect on about 10% of the patients, such as to cause them to live a much longer time. This effect might be such as to "cure" them; that is, to give them the life expectancy that they would have had if they had not developed cancer. On the other hand, it might only set them back one or more stages in the development of the cancer, in which case their life expectancy would be somewhat less than that corresponding to complete elimination of the effect of their having developed cancer. This uncertainty may be eliminated in the course of time, as the survival times of the 18 patients in the ascorbate-treated group who were still living on August 10, 1976 become known.

Conclusion

In this study the times of survival of 100 ascorbate-treated cancer patients in Scotland (measured from the day when the patient was pronounced to have cancer untreatable by conventional methods) have been discussed in comparison with those of 1000 matched controls, 10 for each of the ascorbate-treated patients. The data indicate that deaths occur for about 90% of the ascorbate-treated patients at one third the rate for the controls, so that for this fraction there is a 3-fold increase in survival time, measured from the date when the cancer was pronounced untreatable. For the other 10% of the ascorbate-treated patients the survival time is not known with certainty, but it is indicated by the values in Table 1 to be more than 20 times the average for the untreated patients. The value 4.16 (Table 2) for the ratio of average survival times expresses the resultant of these two effects.

We conclude that there is strong evidence that treatment of patients in Scotland with terminal (untreatable) cancer with about 10 g of ascorbate (ascorbic acid, vitamin C) per day increases the survival time by the factor of about 3 for most of them and by at least 20 for a few (about 10%). It is our opinion that a similar effect would be found for untreatable cancer patients in other countries. Larger amounts than 10 g/day might have a greater effect. Moreover, we surmise that the addition of ascorbate to the treatment of patients with cancer at an earlier stage of development might well have a similar effect, changing life expectancy after the stage when ascorbate treatment is begun from, for example, 5 years to 20 years.

This study was supported by research grants from the Secretary of State for Scotland and The Educational Foundation of America, and by contributions by private donors to the Linus Pauling Institute.

1. Cameron, E. & Pauling, L., "Ascorbic acid and the glycosaminoglycans: An orthomolecular approach to cancer and other diseases," *Oncology*, vol. 27, pp. 181–192, 1973.

2. Cameron, E. & Pauling, L., "The orthomolecular treatment of cancer: I. The role of ascorbic acid in host resistance," *Chemico-Biological Interactions*, pp. 273–283, 1974.

3. Cameron, E., "Biological function of ascorbic acid and the pathogenesis of scurvy: a working hypothesis," *Medical Hypotheses*, vol. 3, pp. 154–163, 1976.

4. Cameron, E. & Campbell, A., "The orthomolecular

treatment of cancer: II. Clinical trial of high-dose ascorbic acid supplements in advanced human cancer," *Chemico-Biological Interactions,* vol. 9, pp. 285–315, 1974.

5. Cameron, E., Campbell, A. & Jack, T., "The ortho-molecular treatment of cancer: III. Reticulum cell sarcoma: double complete regression induced by high-dose ascorbic acid therapy," *Chemico-Biological Interactions,* vol. 11, pp. 387–393, 1975.

Appendix B
The Orthomolecular Treatment of Cancer

The following are brief summaries of three important scientific papers on the theory and use of vitamin C to treat cancer. Anyone wishing copies of the original papers can get them by writing to: The Linus Pauling Institute of Science and Medicine, 2700 Sand Hill Road, Menlo Park California 94025. Since considerable expense is involved in producing reprints such as these, I would suggest that a donation to the institute be made at the time the papers are requested.

I. The Role of Ascorbic Acid in Host Resistance *

By Ewan Cameron and Linus Pauling

For the best possible treatment of cancer many approaches need to be used, including surgery, radiation, chemotherapy, immunotherapy, and nutritional therapy.

Nutritional therapy for cancer patients has been neglected. However, if the patient's natural defense mechanisms against cancer are to be supported to the utmost, ideal nutrition must be given to the cancer patient, including vitamin C.

Cancer cells have been demonstrated in 50 percent of patients undergoing surgery for colon or rectal cancer. Yet this 50 percent had no higher mortality rate from cancer than the 50 percent in whom no cancer cells were found in the blood stream. Obviously the patients' natural resistance killed off these "floating" cancer cells.

---

* Original paper appeared in *Chemico–Biological Interactions*, vol. 9, pp. 273–287, 1974.

Ideal nutrition should help keep people from developing cancer in the first place and, should they get cancer, should help the body fight off the disease.

It has been demonstrated that patients with cancer have low body reserves of vitamin C.

Vitamin C, as well as ideal total nutrition, should help prevent cancer. It should be a valuable supportive treatment when given along with conventional cancer treatments. Vitamin C should be given in large amounts especially to reduce pain, provide a feeling of well being, and prolong the life of terminally ill cancer patients.

II. Clinical Trial of High-Dose Ascorbic Acid Supplements in Advanced Human Cancer *

By Ewan Cameron and Allan Campbell

This study deals with the first fifty patients with terminal cancer who were treated by these men with massive amounts of vitamin C. They give a brief summary of the diagnosis, treatment and outcome of each patient.

To me the most interesting things about the paper are the X-ray pictures illustrating cases 44 and 45.

Case 44 is a fifty-five-year-old man with cancer of the kidney that had spread to the bones. Figure 1 shows an X-ray picture of the upper arm where the cancer has eaten away the bone. Figure 2 shows the same view of the arm 220 days after receiving the vitamin C. In the second picture we see quite clearly that the bone has begun to form again, that the cancer is beginning to fade away.

The hipbone of the same patient showed the same healing process at work 395 days after having the vitamin C treatment.

Figure 3 shows the chest X-ray of case 45, a forty-year-old male with untreated reticulum cell sarcoma that had spread to the chest. Figure 4 shows a perfectly normal chest X ray after the patient had been on vitamin C for 70 days.

---

* Original paper appeared in *Chemico–Biological Interactions*, vol. 9, pp. 285–315, 1974.

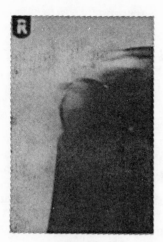

FIG. 1

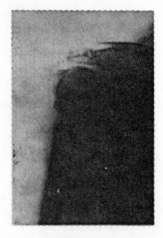

FIG. 2

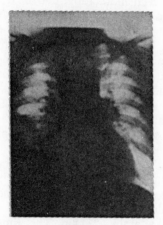

FIG. 3

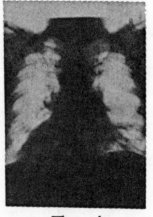

FIG. 4

III. Reticulum Cell Sarcoma: Double Complete Regression Induced by High-Dose Ascorbic Acid Therapy *

By Ewan Cameron, Allan Campbell, and Thomas Jack

This is a detailed study of the patient mentioned in the previous paper—case 45, a forty-year-old man who entered the hospital and was diagnosed as having a reticulum cell sarcoma. A chest X ray revealed extensive involvement of the right lung. Physical examination showed that he had an enlarged liver and spleen. Many large rubbery lymph nodes were present in the neck. Diagnosis was established by biopsy.

He could not be transferred at once to a hospital specialized in treating cancer with chemotherapy, and in the meantime was started on large doses of vitamin C.

Within ten days of starting the vitamin C therapy the patient's appetite returned, he lost his weakness and night sweats, and he felt like a new man. Chest X ray at the end of fourteen days of treatment showed clearing. His liver and spleen returned to normal size.

Two and a half months after beginning vitamin C therapy (he had no other treatment) his chest X ray was completely clear and there were no physical signs of illness. He felt well and returned to work.

Some four months later, after gradually reducing the vitamin C and then leaving it off completely for a month, he returned to the hospital complaining of tiredness and a cough. A chest X ray revealed a return of the cancer.

The patient was started on vitamin C again. This time his improvement was slower, but gradually he lost all of his symptoms. At the end of seven months a chest X ray showed his lungs had again cleared completely.

---

* Original paper appeared in *Chemico–Biological Interactions*, vol. 11, pp. 387–393, 1975.

Notes

Chapter 15: A Modern-Day Horror Story
1. Carl C. Pfeiffer, *Zinc and Other Micro-Nutrients* (New Canaan, Conn.: Keats Publishing, Inc., 1978).

Chapter 17: Diet
1. *Medical Tribune,* November 17, 1976.
J. H. Weisburger et al., "Colon Cancer: Its Epidemiology and Experimental Production," *Cancer,* vol. 40, no. 5, November 1977.
E. L. Wynder et al. in *Cancer Detection and Prevention* (New York: Marcel Dekker, Inc., 1977).
2. P. Correa, W. Haenszel, C. Cuello, et al., *Lancet,* vol. 2, p. 58, 1975.
W. Haenszel and P. Correa, *Cancer Research,* vol. 35, p. 3452, 1975.
T. Hirayama, *Cancer Research,* vol. 35, p. 3460, 1975.
H. Marquardt, F. Rufino, and J. H. Weisburger, *Food and Cosmetics Toxicology,* vol. 15, p. 97, 1977.
H. Marquardt, F. Rufino, and J. H. Weisburger, *Science,* vol. 196, p. 1000, 1977.
S. S. Mirvish, *Annals of the New York Academy of Science,* vol 258, p. 175, 1975.
S. S. Mirvish, L. Wallcave, M. Eagen, and P. Shubik, *Science,* vol. 177, p. 65, 1972.
R. Raineri and J. H. Weisburger, *Science,* vol. 177, p. 181, 1972.
J. H. Weisburger, "Vitamin C and Prevention of Nitrosamine Formation," *Lancet* (September 17, 1977).

3. Richard Passwater, *Supernutrition for Healthy Hearts* (New York: The Dial Press, 1977).

4. Robert Ardrey, *The Hunting Hypothesis* (New York: Atheneum Publishers, 1976).

5. D. and P. Brothwell, *Food in Antiquity* (New York: Praeger Publishers, Inc., 1969).

6. Linus Pauling, *Vitamin C, the Common Cold and the Flu* (San Francisco: W. H. Freeman & Company Publishers, 1976), p. 194.

Chapter 20: Vitamins and Minerals to Prevent Cancer

1. J. W. McCormick, *Archives of Pediatrics* (October 1954).

2. Linus Pauling, *Vitamin C, the Common Cold and the Flu* (San Francisco: W. H. Freeman & Company Publishers, San Francisco, 1976), p. 194.

3. P. Correa, W. Haenszel, C. Cuello, et al., *Lancet,* vol. 2, p. 58, 1975.

4. T. Hirayama, *Cancer Research,* vol. 35, p. 3460, 1975.

5. W. Haenszel and P. Correa, *Cancer Research,* vol. 35, p. 3452, 1975.

6. H. Marquardt, F. Rufino, and J. H. Weisburger, *Science,* vol. 196, p. 1000, 1977.

7. H. Marquardt, F, Rufino, and J. H. Weisburger, *Food and Cosmetics Toxicology,* vol. 15, p. 97, 1977.

8. S. S. Mirvish, *Annals of the New York Academy of Science,* vol. 258, p. 175, 1975.

9. S. S. Mirvish, L. Wallcave, M. Eagen, and P. Shubik, *Science,* vol. 177, p. 65, 1972.

10. L. Poirier, *Medical Tribune* p. 9, November 17, 1976.

11. R. Raineri and J. H. Weisburger, *Annals of the New York Academy of Science,* vol. 258, p. 181, 1975.

12. J. H. Weisburger, "Vitamin C and Prevention of Nitrosamine Formation," *Lancet,* September 17, 1977.

13. P. Rous, "The Virus Tumors and the Tumor Problem," Harvey Lecture, 1935.

14. C. W. Jungeblut, "Inactivation of Poliomyelitis Virus by Crystalline Ascorbic Acid," *Journal of Experimental Medicine,* vol. 62, pp. 517–21, 1935.

15. G. Amato, "Azione Dellacido Ascorbico sul Virus Fisso Della Rabbia e sulla Tossina Tetancia," *Giornale di*

Bacteriologica, Virologia et Immunologia (Torino), vol. 19, pp. 843–49, 1937.

16. T. W. Anderson et al., "Vitamin C and the Common Cold: A Double Blind Clinical Trial," *Journal of Canadian Medical Association,* vol. 107, pp. 503–508, 1972.

17. H. Bauer, "Poliomyelitis Therapy with Ascorbic Acid," *Helvetica Medica Acta,* vol. 19, pp. 470–74. 1952.

18. O. Gsell et al., "Treatment of Epidemic Poliomyelitis with High Doses of Ascorbic Acid," *Schweizersche Medizinische Wochenshrift,* vol. 84, pp. 661–66, 1954.

19. M. Holden et al., "In Vitro Action of Synthetic Crystalline Vitamin C (Asocrbic Acid) on Herpes Virus," *Journal of Immunology,* vol. 31, pp. 455–62, 1936.

20. F. R. Klenner, "The Treatment of Poliomyelitis and Other Virus Diseases with Vitamin C," *Southern Medicine and Surgery,* vol. 3, pp. 209–14, 1949.

21. I. J. Kligler et al., "Inactivation of Vaccina Virus By Ascorbic Acid and Glutathione," *Nature,* vol. 13a, pp. 965–66, 1937.

22. W. Langenbusch et al., "Einfluss der Vitamine auf das Virus der Maul-und Klauenseuch," *Zentral Blatt fur Backteriologie,* vol. 140, pp. 112–15, 1937.

23. M. Lojkin, *Contributions of the Joyce Thompson Institute,* vol. 8, p. 4, 1936. L. E. Martin, *Proceedings Third International Congress of Microbiology, New York, 1940,* p. 281.

24. A. B. Savin, "Vitamin C in Relation to Experimental Poliomyelitis," *Journal of Experimental Medicine,* vol. 69, pp. 507–15, 1939.

25. L. Benade, T. Howard, and D. Burk, "Synergistic Killing of Ehrlich Ascites Carcinoma Cells by Ascorbic and 3-Amino-1, 2, 4-Triazole," *Oncology,* vol. 23, pp. 33–43, 1969.

26. J. A. Kalden et al., "Prolonged Skin Allograft Survival in Vitamin C Deficient Guinea Pigs," *European Surgical Research,* vol. 4, pp. 114–19, 1972.

27. P. Issenberg, "Nitrite, Nitrosamines and Cancer," *Federal Proceedings,* vol. 35, p. 1322, 1976.

28. M. Rustia, "Inhibitory Effect of Sodium Ascorbate on Ethylurea and Sodium Nitrite Carcinogenesis and Negative Findings in Progeny after Inoculation of Precursors

into Pregnant Hamsters," *Journal of the National Cancer Institute*, vol. 55, p. 1389, 1975.

29. J. V. Schlegel et al., "The Role of Ascorbic Acid in the Prevention of Bladder Tumor Formation," *Journal of Urology*, vol. 103, p. 155, 1970.

30. P. W. A. Mansell et al., *Journal of the National Cancer Institute*, vol. 54, p. 571, 1975.

31. M. V. Cone et al., *Journal of the National Cancer Institute*, vol. 50, p. 1599, 1973.

32. N. H. Rowe et al., *Cancer*, vol. 26, p. 436, 1970.

33. M. B. Sporn et al., *Federal Proceedings*, vol. 35, p. 1332, 1976.

34. R. J. Shamberger, *Journal of the National Cancer Institute*, vol. 47, p. 667, 1971.

35. H. F. Kraybill, *Clinical Pharmacology and Therapeutics*, January and February, 1963.

36. R. Willhern et al., *Gastroenterology*, vol. 23, 1953, and *Nutritional Review*, vol. 4, p. 353, 1946.

37. L. A. Cerkes et al., *Nutrition Abstracts and Reviews*, vol. 30, p. 955, 1960.

38. J. R. Davidson, *Journal of the Canadian Medical Association*, vol. 31, p. 486, 1934.

39. D. B. Carter, *Path. Bact.*, vol. 63, p. 599, 1951.

40. C. G. Tedeschi, *Archives of Pathology*, vol. 47, p. 160, 1949.

Chapter 23: Detailed Instructions for the Use of Massive Amounts of Vitamin C in the Treatment of Cancer

1. H. L. Newbold, "Relationship Between Spontaneous Allergic Conditions and Ascorbic Acid," *Journal of Allergy*, vol. 15, p. 385, November 1944.

2. St. Rusznyak and A. Szent-Györgyi, *Nature*, vol. 138, p. 27, 1936.

3. Armentano, Bentsath, Beres, et al., *Deutsche Medizinische Wochenschrift*, vol. 62, p. 1325, 1936.

4. Z. Zlock, *International Journal of Vitamin Research*, vol. 39, p. 269, 1969.

5. M. E. Shils and R. S. Goodhardt, *The Flavonoids in Biology and Medicine* (New York: The National Vitamin Foundation, 1956).

Chapter 24: Are Large Amounts of Vitamin C Toxic?

1. T. W. Anderson et al., *Journal of the Canadian Medical Association*, vol. 111, pp. 31–36, 1974.

J. L. Coulehan et al., *New England Journal of Medicine*, vol. 290, pp. 6–10, 1974.

T. Gordonoff, *Schweizerische Medizinische Wochenschrift*, vol. 90, pp. 726–29, 1960.

A. Hoffer, *Lancet*, p. 1146, November 17, 1973.

N. Jakowlew, *Ernaebruns Forschung*, vol. 3, pp. 446–47, 1958.

W. J. Rhead and G. N. Schrauzer, *Nutrition Reviews*, vol. 29, pp. 262–63, 1971.

2. H. H. Hutchins, P. J. Cravioto, and T. J. Macek, *Journal of the American Pharmocology Association*, vol. 45, pp. 806–808, 1956. See also V. Herbert and E. Jacob, *Journal of the American Medical Association*, vol. 230, no. 2, pp. 241–42, 1974.

3. H. L. Newmark, J. Scheiner, and M. Marcus, *American Journal of Clinical Nutrition*, vol. 29, pp. 645–49, 1976.

4. S. Lewin, *Vitamin C: Its Molecular Biology and Medical Potential* (New York: Academic Press, 1976).

5. E. P. Samborskaya and T. D. Ferdman, *Bjulletin Eksperimentalnoi Biologii i Meditsinii*, vol. 62, pp. 96–98, 1966.